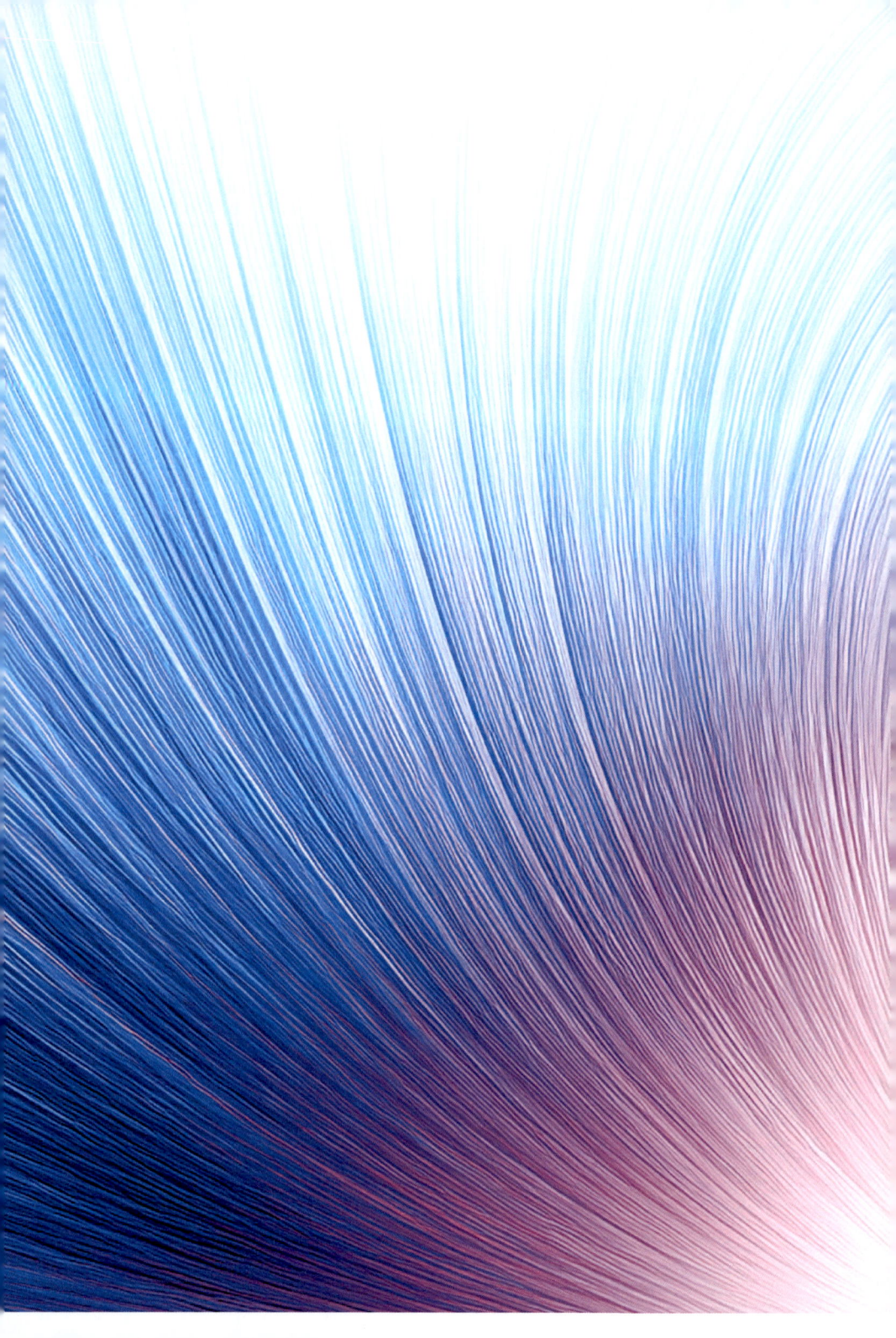

Independently published
Writer: Lee Jones
Cover & interior design: Laura Reid, ChatGPT
First Edition – 2025

UNBOXED

Stop eating fake, start eating real
A no-nonsense guide to
additive-free living

By Lee Jones

The beginning I didn't see coming

I thought it was the end — but it was the start of everything that finally made sense.

You don't notice when your world starts to blur — not at first. You just keep pushing, working, fixing, surviving. Until one day, the mask slips, and you realise it's not you that's broken... it's the system you've been trying to fit into. That was my beginning. The one I didn't see coming.

I've always felt a bit different.

Not in a bad way — just different.

Like my brain was wired to notice things others didn't. Even as a kid, I could take apart a bike and rebuild it, remember how something worked just by glancing at it, or spot problems others missed.

My dad saw this in me early on — I got it from him.

He's a short guy — about 5'3", bald on top, with a bit of a pot belly — but he's got this warmth about him. He was always doing something, and if he wasn't, he was on his computer in his room, which was always at the heart of the house. He could do what he loved, right next to his family.

He always let me get involved when he was working. His patience was better than mine. I'd pass him tools and eventually try things myself. I remember being about four years old, sitting cross-legged in the garage, fascinated by the way he could fix anything — **knowing I'd do that too one day.**

By the time I was a teenager, I wasn't just watching — I was installing complex alarm systems on motorbikes, repairing and servicing, working Saturdays, and earning a decent income. I was still just a lad, on £20 a week pocket money, but getting £50 a day on weekends felt like gold.

At first, I was the local sweetshop's best customer — Jason's (if you lived in Moreton in the '80s, you'll know him). But I quickly started saving, all of which was kept in my dad's work safe. Soon, I was buying my own little projects. Dad helped too — sometimes taking bikes in part-exchange or buying one outright using money he'd tucked away for me.

I'd come home from school and he'd say, "I bought this for you," and hand me the keys.

What can a teenager really do with £70 a week?

Strip it, fix it, and bring it back to life.

I was great with a tin of matte black paint, a wire brush, and some basic frame paints. If it needed figuring out, I was in my element.

The only bit I wasn't great at yet was painting and repairing fairings and tanks. But my focus was relentless. I had to know how to do it — and do it properly. Eventually, that turned into another income stream: weekend repairs on bike fairings and small car panels for cash.

But I struggled with school.

Not because I wasn't capable — I just couldn't force my brain to care about things that didn't feel real or useful. I needed challenge, creativity, and purpose. Without that, I switched off.

Even English didn't hold me. I respected Shakespeare for the history, but I couldn't get into it. I wasn't a natural writer. Half the time, I couldn't even read my own handwriting. That just wasn't how my brain worked.

Still, I was polite. I took part when I could. I didn't want to be a nuisance or set a bad example. And funnily enough, my English teacher is now my mother-in-law — and a brilliant grandparent to our kids. Maybe some part of me always knew what was right. I just had to listen to it.

Music and machinery saved me in those years. However, it also included a few wrong turns.

There was a time when I got pulled into the buzz of going out — music, mates, and drugs that made you feel unstoppable. It didn't last long, but it could have.

One night at 16, I ended up in the hospital with heart issues after taking something I shouldn't have.

A nurse took me aside while my mum waited outside. She looked me dead in the eye and said, "If you carry on like this, you won't be here much longer."

She didn't know me.

But she saw me.

And she saw what I'd done.

I was ashamed that day. I pulled myself back together.

Never touched that stuff again.

Cannabis? That stuck around.

I didn't know why it helped me unwind — just that it did. Later, I got into motocross — a movement that demands focus and adrenaline. That saved me differently. I loved the weekends, the technical trails in Wales, the smell of the dirt. I wasn't into causing trouble — I just needed something to be part of. Something to challenge me.

My dad gave me skills. My mum gave me structure. She was the most organised person I knew. Washing done, food prepped, and the house is spotless. I didn't realise until later how much that mattered. **How important it is to have a safe place to come home to.**

A place to breathe when life feels like too much.

That foundation shaped me — and when things got messy, I always craved that same sense of calm.

Opening Chapter - Part 2

The Turning Point

After school, I chased a few things. College, bodywork, my own shop. I was ambitious and driven, constantly seeking new challenges. Relationships, business ventures, fatherhood — all of it came fast, sometimes too fast. I became a dad young. I built businesses, bought property, made good money, lost it, and started again.

On paper, I had success.

But inside? I often felt misunderstood, overwhelmed, and like I was running on fumes.

Everything changed the day my firstborn son arrived.

That moment hit different — like life zoomed out and I could finally see what actually mattered. He gave me purpose. A reason to be better.

A reason to get up, to graft, to fix what felt broken. All the stuff I'd been chasing before suddenly seemed small.

I'd look at him and feel this mix of fear, pride, and love so deep it made me want to fight harder — for him, and for the version of me he deserved to grow up with.

I look back now, and although it was challenging and busy, I was going somewhere — financially.

I had a son and something that looked good from the outside.

But no one saw the difficult times, the hard work, the long hours.

I can't forget them.

He was — and still is — a dream kid. Sixteen now, as I write this.

We split when he was three. I won't go into detail about his mum, but there was no co-parenting, no updates, no shared care. Just silence — like another way to make me feel like I was the one who failed. But I never gave up. I stayed in contact with him. He's always been my boy, and the bond we've got has never been shaken. No matter what's said or not said around it all, I believe the truth always shows in time.

And even if it doesn't — I still did the right thing.

That's one of my core values.

Opening Chapter - Part 3

Finding Jen

Soon after the split, I found myself floating.

I've never been one for social media — it's never felt real to me — but life has a funny way of putting things in front of you when you least expect it. I was sitting with my dad one day, going over what to do next, feeling a bit lost. A few days had passed, and I just wandered, wondering what life was trying to tell me.

Then a moment came.

I was scrolling through my phone, and a suggested friend popped up.

Jen.

My Jen. From school.

We'd kind of had a thing back then — young fire, that unspoken spark. Jen used to wear my coat in school. I liked that. She had someone older interested in her too, but I never cared. I've never been afraid of going after what I want. I think this book proves that.

Then, just like that, she was gone. Her mum moved them down south after Year 10 — and with her went the "what if" that lingered for years.

So, there I was, heart thumping over a bloody Facebook notification.

I had to message. But what do you even say?

I think I typed something like: "Hello… long time no see."

Cringey, but honest.

To be fair, it was more than curiosity. I was going through a divorce, so yeah — messy, and maybe a bit much for most people. But deep down, I already knew what my gut was telling me. And when I truly listen to my gut, it's never wrong.

So, I sent the message...

It turned out that Jen was living in Huddersfield, finishing university. She'd been in Greece for years, had many stories, and belonged to a close-knit group of friends she loved like family.

From the first message… it just clicked.

We talked non-stop. The only time we stopped messaging was when we were together. I was persistent — I'd have driven up that night if she let me — but she made me wait just long enough.

And when we finally met again, I knew.

That gut feeling? It said, "This is home".

Opening Chapter - Part 4

Building Something Real

Huddersfield gave me more than just Jen.

I made real friends for the first time since I was in school. Not just people to hang around with — people who got me.

Jon was one of them — sharp, funny, structured, and gym-obsessed like me. His mate Mike, too. They welcomed me like a brother. We don't talk much now — maybe it's an ADHD thing, perhaps just life — but when we do, it's like nothing's changed.

It felt like home…

I had a short career working for others — a bit of a love-hate thing, really.

Take Car sales, for example.

I had a few jobs while living in Huddersfield, but working as a new car sales exec was the most… character-building. The usual dealership pressure was there: targets, endless KPIs, office politics — all of it.

Then there was the business manager.

Our relationship? Classic ADHD-meets-corporate-misfit. He moaned about everything — the seat wasn't quite right, the mirror had moved, the fuel light was on. God forbid you took his demonstrator out for more than three minutes without a full tank and a valeting session.

Always the same speech: "Put £20 in, don't touch the seat, don't touch the mirrors, and make sure it's hoovered."

Blah blah blah.

I treated that like a 'what not to do' list.

Late one Sunday, showroom dead quiet, my brain buzzing as usual. A family walked in and ended up test-driving a car — funnily enough, almost identical spec to his precious company car.

Impulse kicked in.

After the drive, I tipped a whole load of hole punch dots into his air vents.

Like confetti for corporate pettiness.

Next morning — dashboard like a snow globe in a wind tunnel.

Few of the lads knew — even the used car manager and his brother. They saw the funny side.

It was childish, sure. But in my head, it felt… worth it.

That was ADHD humour in action — reward first, deal with later.

Then came the new sales manager.

Clipboard energy. Four-piece suit, two sizes too tight.

All motivational quotes and late night cold-call schemes.

He told me, "We're calling leads from 6–8 pm. It's part of the job. Trust me."

I said, "Yeah… I won't be doing that."

Still stayed late — out of principle, not submission — but didn't make a single call.

Then came the idea.

He'd recently been eyeing up an Audi. A friend tipped me off and provided some statistics to work with. So, I rang him that evening from my personal mobile; he didn't know the number, pretending to be from Audi's new lead team.

"Hi there — just following up on your recent interest in the A5…"

He answered, snappy and annoyed.

"I've just walked in the house. I don't appreciate being called during family time."

I apologised and said it was part of a new follow-up initiative — one that only targets interested buyers.

He bit. Said it was disrespectful. Poor timing. Unprofessional.

Perfect.

He didn't clock it was me until the next meeting… when I brought it up.

I could see the penny drop.

Didn't say a word — just gave me the look.

He pulled me aside.

Told me I wasn't a team player.

Said I was the reason it "wasn't working."

I told him, "If someone's genuinely interested, they'll come to you." "You're burning their customers with your amateurish efforts."

Didn't go down well. I was soon sat in front of HR, and gone the same day…

To be honest, we had plans anyway. We were off to Greece, and soon after, moving to the Wirral.

I popped back in one day to tie things up — turns out the car manager role was open.

It always baffled me how companies look outward for roles that they already have someone qualified for in-house. Loyalty overlooked. Skills wasted.

However, I still wish him well.

I genuinely hoped he learned something from it.

Opening Chapter - Part 5

The Wedding & What Came After

Then came the wedding.

We got married at Peckforton Castle — a dream setting that felt straight out of a storybook. Jon was my best man. Mike was there. A few others who mattered.

It was magical. But it didn't come without stress.

Planning a castle wedding while juggling life's chaos should've broken us — but it didn't.

We made it work with family support, sheer graft, and madness.

The pressure was enormous. But the day? Perfect.

I was on cloud nine — surrounded by love, laughter, and the kind of atmosphere that makes you stop and feel lucky to be alive.

Then came the Maldives. Our honeymoon.

Calm, peaceful, the break I didn't know I needed.

We got back. Moved into a new house on the Wirral.

And I landed the job that would shape the next chapter of my life.

Opening Chapter - Part 6

The Bodyshop & Finding My Place

I started on the tools, panel beating. Then, I moved into estimating.

The team there weren't just coworkers — they were like cousins. And then there was James.

My manager. My mate.

He was the first leader — outside of my dad — who really got me.

Calm. Observant. Fair. James gave direction like my dad — anchored, no drama. But with banter and belief that made you want to be better.

I looked forward to work. I felt seen. Respected.

The Body Shop was voted best in the UK by many prestigious

manufacturers. The team earned that, and James made it.

James was soon promoted. New adventure in the same company. To do what James does best...

I knew the place wouldn't be the same. And I was right.

Things shifted. Decisions got made by people who didn't know the team like he did. The wrong person got promoted. The team was disrupted. Morale dropped.

Eventually, I left, too.

But I never forgot what that job — and James — gave me.

It wasn't just a wage.

It was one of the few places in my life that ever felt like belonging.

I thought we'd catch up again one day.

Tell him what I'd been through. How it all hit the fan. How I burned out. How I clawed it back.
But then the call came.

Opening Chapter - Part 7

The Call That Changed Everything

James had passed away.

A skydiving accident.

2024.
When I heard, it knocked the wind out of me.

I never got to thank him. I never got to tell him that he reminded me of the man I used to be — the one I was trying to find again.

He was calm, steady, and sharp. A rare kind of leader. And more than that — he was my mate.

I hope he knew how much people respected him. I still think about his family and his partner, Chloe. They shared that skydiving world with a close group of friends as well. I hope she still feels him with her at every jump.

I know he would. Probably up to mischief, too, knowing him.

I even did a jump once, for a charity event for The Body Shop.

Jen wasn't so sure, but she supported me. It's a core memory now. One I'll always keep.

I have the video still. Maybe I'll share it one day. He recorded it and jumped with me.

I still struggle to watch it if I'm honest.

Some memories scar you. Some shape you.

This one did both. Especially now anyway...

Opening Chapter - Part 8

The Diagnosis That Made Everything Click

In March 2023, I was diagnosed with ADHD.

It was a shock.

I'd spent months in therapy, tried antidepressants, pushed through burnout — and still felt off.

My understanding of ADHD was old-school: fidgety kids, not grown men running businesses and raising families. But when I started digging, it hit like a freight train.

Everything made sense.

The highs. The crashes. The chaos. The cannabis. The cravings. The hyperfocus. The overwhelm.

I wasn't broken.

I was wired differently.

I studied like mad. Hyperfocus kicked in. I had to know.

And with every layer I uncovered, I began to see the world — and myself — more clearly.

But I still didn't feel fully myself.

Something was still off.

Then came a virus. Just a flu, I thought.

Cold sweats. No appetite. Blurry vision. Heart racing. My meds weren't working — if anything, they were making it worse.

So, I took a weekend off. No meds. Just rest, clean food, and time with my family.

Saturday morning, I was up at 6. Normally, I'd be straight on the medication. But this time, I left it.

By the time I was 7, I'd made breakfast for the kids. Poached eggs on toast. Simple. Decent.

We went out as a family — nothing fancy. Just a walk to the park, some fresh air, and a bit for tea.

I noticed something... I felt lighter.

Later that day, we built a den in the living room, right in front of the telly.

The kids loved it. I used to love that as a kid, too.

It was the first time in years the TV wasn't even on. And I didn't miss it.

After bath time, we made dinner, put the kids to bed, and sat out in the garden — just me and Jen.

I fell asleep by half nine. Deep, uninterrupted sleep. The kind that hugs your soul.

Sunday morning, I woke before my alarm.

And for the first time in what felt like forever, I didn't feel broken.

I felt… peaceful.

That was the moment I knew.

Something in me had changed.

So, I started writing.

Not because I wanted to — but because I had to. I needed to get the past out of my head. I needed to understand it.

And I needed to figure out why I felt better that weekend than I had in years.

I created two lists: one for my diet that week and another for what I typically eat.

And that's when I saw it.

The additives.

The sugar.

The chemicals are in everything — food, drink, water.

I was living in survival mode. Eating crap. Sleeping badly. Running on fumes.

And all those additives? They were stripping me of clarity, energy, focus, joy.

My medication hadn't stopped working.

My body had started healing.

And now?

I take a much lower dose.

I eat better.

I sleep more deeply.

And my brain — the one I thought was broken — is coming back to life.

Opening Chapter - Part 9

Where Unboxed Begins

So, this is where Unboxed begins.

Not in a lab.

Not in a TikTok.

Not in a lecture from someone who's never lived it.

But in a kitchen.

On a sofa.

In a moment of stillness, where I could finally hear myself think.

I'm just a lad from the Wirral who grew up in the '80s. And this journey was given to me for a reason.

Because I would have to figure it out.

I couldn't let it go.

And I would find myself again — even if it nearly killed me.

The system profits from us being too exhausted to question it.

This book isn't about being perfect.

It's not a diet plan.

It's not a conspiracy theory.

And it's not just for people with ADHD.

It's for anyone who's felt foggy, exhausted, forgotten, fed up, or numb — like I was.

But here's the thing:

We always have the choice to fight.

Not just out there — but in here.

To take back our clarity.

Our focus.

Our lives.

So, this is my story.

But it's also your story.

Because the world doesn't need more perfect people.

It needs more of you — unboxed.

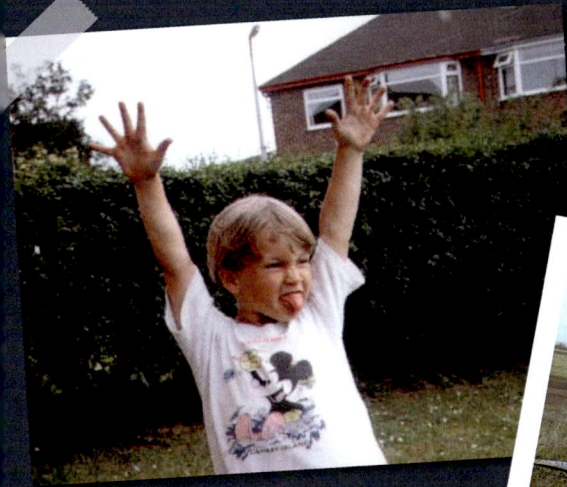
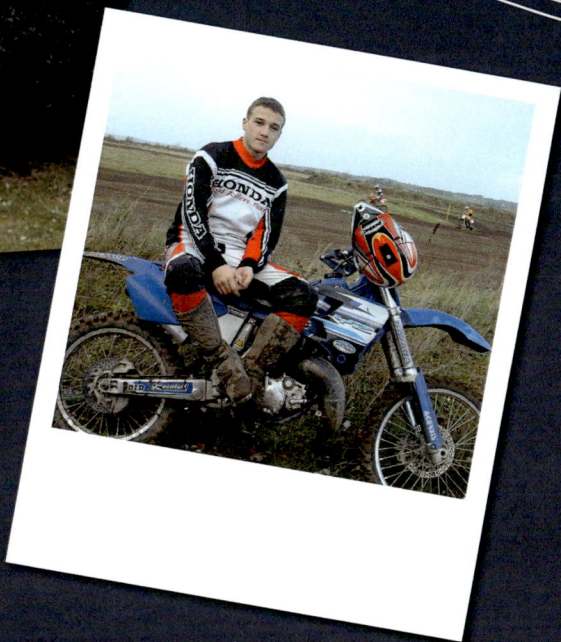
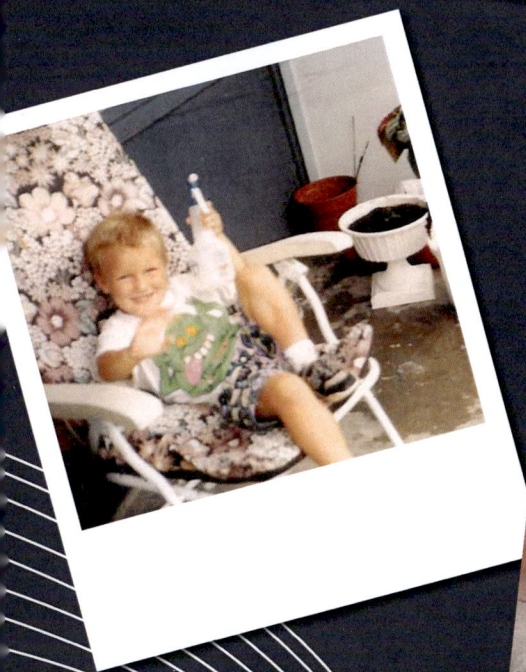
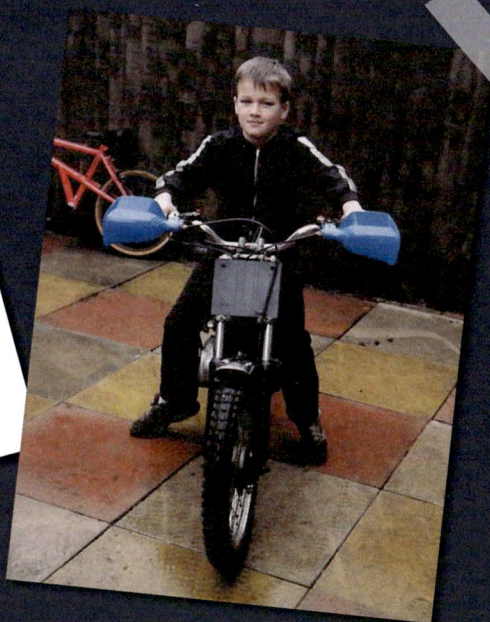

Chapter 1 - Part 1

What's Really in Our Food?

I used to think food was food.

If it was on the shelves, it must be safe, right?

I didn't grow up questioning labels or wondering what those tiny E-numbers meant. I was more interested in what tasted good — like everyone else. But looking back now, I realise how much trust I was placing in the system. **And how wrong that trust turned out to be.**

Most of us are unaware of what's in the food we eat every day.

Not really.

We scan the front of the packet — "low fat," "high in fibre," "natural flavours" — and assume we're doing okay. But turn it over, and the back tells a very different story.

Chemical names. Preservatives. Colours. Acids. Artificial sweeteners.

And worst of all, many of these aren't just unnecessary... they're harmful, especially to our brains.

The Silent Ingredients

You don't need to be allergic to have a reaction to something. Some things don't cause rashes or swelling — they cause irritability, brain fog, mood swings, hyperactivity, or crashes that feel like burnout.

And if you're already someone with ADHD, anxiety, depression, or other neurodivergent traits?

You're likely more sensitive, not less.

But here's the thing: these sensitivities are almost always ignored. They don't show up on a blood test. They don't trigger a panic from doctors. And they don't seem like "real" problems — until you realise, they've been chipping away at your energy, focus, and mood for years.

Chapter 1 - Part 2

My Wake-Up Call

It wasn't a sudden event that made me question it. It was a gradual awareness — a moment here, a clue there — until I couldn't ignore it any longer.

At first, I noticed how different I felt after certain meals.

Then it was spotting patterns: the crashes after energy drinks, the short fuse after certain sweets, the restless nights after a "treat tea."

It got louder after I started medication for ADHD. Suddenly, I had a clearer baseline. I felt the difference more acutely. Days when I'd eaten better? Calmer. Sharper. More emotionally present.

Days I didn't? I was overwhelmed by midday.

Eventually, I did what most people never do: I started reading the labels.

Not just glancing — really reading. And researching. And logging how I felt.

The Hidden Triggers

Here are some of the additives I started spotting everywhere:

E220 (Sulphur dioxide) – in dried fruits and wine, linked to headaches and behaviour shifts.

E621 (MSG) – a flavour enhancer that can overstimulate the brain's glutamate receptors.

E129 (Allura Red) – found in yoghurts, soft drinks, linked to hyperactivity in kids.

Aspartame – an artificial sweetener that messed with my mood and gave me tension headaches.

These weren't rare chemicals. They were in my kitchen, my kids' lunchboxes, my trusted "healthy" brands, and even in medication.

I had no idea how much crap I was putting into my body — and worse, how it was amplifying my ADHD symptoms.

"It's Just a Bit of Sugar"

That's what people say.

Or "It's fine in small amounts."

But what if you're eating "small amounts" of 12 different synthetic compounds... every day?

There's no real testing for that.

No long-term studies on what happens to neurodivergent kids drinking synthetic dyes, eating processed cereal, chewing on sweeteners, and taking medications loaded with binders and colourants.

We assume the system's watching out for us.

It's not.

Chapter 1 - Part 3

The Straw That Broke the Label

One day, I found myself scanning a fruit drink that claimed to be "100% natural." The front showed berries, a sunrise, and a wholesome smiley logo.

The ingredients?

• Water
• Fruit juice from concentrate
• Flavourings
• Citric acid
• Sucralose
• Colour (E163)

That wasn't food. It was a brand exercise.

That's when it clicked: I'd been eating stories, not nourishment.

I started purging the cupboards. Not in a panicked way — just calmly. Reading. Researching. Noticing.

And replacing.

Not everything overnight — but one swap at a time.

The Truth They Don't Advertise

No one's going to shout about how their strawberry yoghurt is actually white, dyed red with synthetic chemicals.

No one's going to tell you your cereal bar contains more chemical energy than nutrition.

Because they can't. If we really knew what we were buying, we wouldn't be buying it anymore.

And that? That would cost them billions.

My Mission Changed

This isn't about fear. It's about clarity.

I don't want people panicking at the supermarket — I want them empowered.

Able to scan a label and think, "Nah, not worth it."

To know the swaps that work. The brands that care. The choices that heal.

Because once you see it, you can't unsee it.

And once you taste absolute clarity… You never want to go back to fog.

Key Takeaway:

"It's not what we eat occasionally that harms us — it's what we feed ourselves daily without questioning."

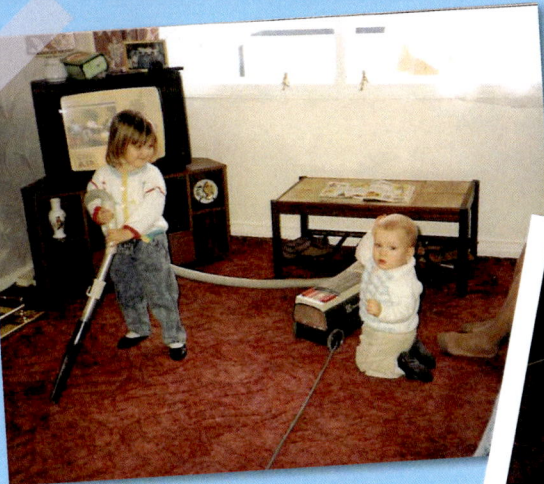

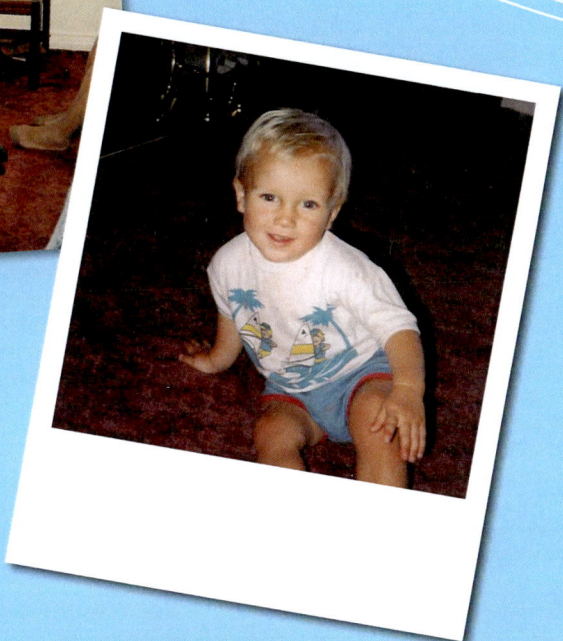

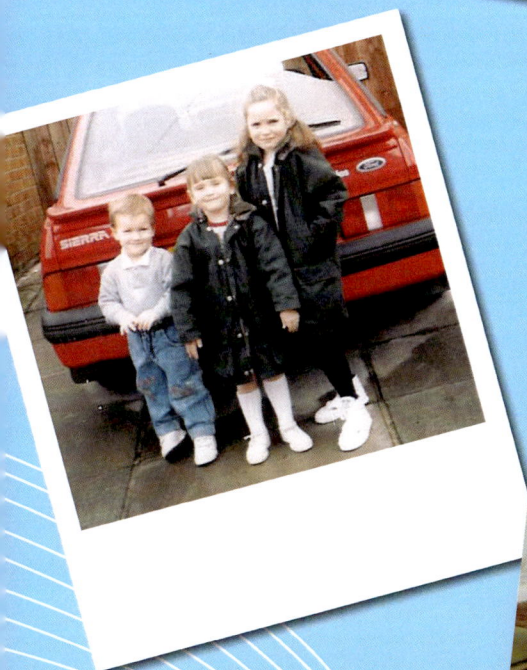

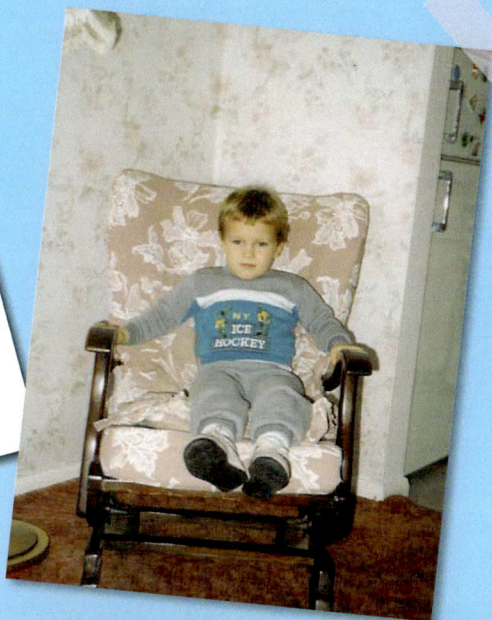

Chapter 2 - Part 1

The Fog We Call Normal

Most people don't realise they're in a fog... until they emerge from it.

You wake up tired. You snap at someone. You can't think straight, so you scroll. You overeat. Then crash. Then reach for caffeine. You drag your mind to focus — and when it won't, you call yourself lazy, broken, unmotivated.

But what if that fog — that constant almost — wasn't your fault?

What if it were chemical?

What if it was coming from your kitchen, not your character?

Waking Up from the Wrong Normal

After starting ADHD medication, I experienced what I can only describe as mental clarity. For the first time, I could think straight. I wasn't constantly battling my own mind just to do basic tasks.

But then something shifted.

I'd found my correct dose — 70mg, the highest for this particular medication. It helped, no doubt. But after a virus, some family stress, and feeling burnt out, I took a break — both from work and from the meds.

That week, we also decided to eat healthier as a family. Clean meals. No processed stuff. More watcr. Real food. I wasn't expecting much — just a bit more energy, maybe.

But what I got… was clarity.

By the weekend, I felt like a different person.

A Weekend That Changed Everything

Saturday morning. No meds. No energy drinks. Just a good breakfast and time with the kids.

By 6:30 am, when I'd typically be waiting for the medication to kick in, I already felt sharp. My patience was back. My thoughts were calm. I wasn't on edge. I wasn't overstimulated. I wasn't… tired.

It felt like me.

Not a high. Not a crash. Just clear.

That day stands out as one of my favourites ever.

I felt alive, present, balanced — without the meds.

I had to understand why.

Chapter 2 - Part 2

Connecting the Dots

That night, I began comparing the ingredients — what I had eaten before and what I was eating now. I started digging into additives. Googling E-numbers. Side effects. Scientific papers. Forums.

E127 (Erythrosine) stood out first. Linked to behavioural shifts. Banned in some countries.

Then E211. Aspartame. Artificial colourings. Preservatives. Sweeteners I couldn't pronounce. Even some of my meds.

I'd always assumed my fog was ADHD. That it was my brain. But now, it seemed... it might've been my environment. My food. My habits. Even the medication — at that strength — might have been masking the real issue.

A Call That Confirmed It

Monday, I took the meds again.

By 8:00 a.m., the fog had returned. Headache. Anxiety. Shaky hands. I rang the doctor.

We went through everything: my symptoms, my diet shift, my weekend off meds. He told me my heart rate was unusually high, my system was overstimulated, and the dose was likely too strong.

He arranged a reduced dosage — but I knew by then it wasn't just about the meds.

The food had amplified everything.

A Massage and a Massive Realisation

The next day, still off meds, I hit the gym and booked a massage — my body felt sore, but my mind was at peace.

That evening, I wrote everything down.

Not just food. But symptoms. Triggers. Ingredients. I went back through a decade of habits in my head — the energy drinks, the late-night snacks, the cereal, the "healthy" products that weren't.

The fog wasn't ADHD alone.

It was a cocktail of fake food, chronic stress, overmedication, and a body that never got the chance to breathe.

The Invisible Additives That Cloud Our Minds

Here are just a few culprits I found:

Aspartame, Acesulfame K – artificial sweeteners, linked to mood swings, tension headaches.

E211 (Sodium Benzoate) – preservative affecting behaviour and focus.

E129, E110 – synthetic colours, linked to hyperactivity.

High Fructose Corn Syrup (HFCS) – disrupts blood sugar, dopamine, and satiety.

These aren't rare. They're in yoghurts, cereals, bread, sauces — even medications. They don't come with warning labels. But they impact your brain daily.

Common Isn't Normal

Needing caffeine to speak in the morning isn't normal.

Crashing after lunch isn't normal.

Brain fog, bloat, anxiety… none of this is normal.

It's just common.

And the more common it becomes, the harder it is to see it clearly.

Small Swaps, Big Shifts

Here are a few swaps that changed everything for me:

Fizzy drinks ⟶ Filtered water or herbal tea

Cereal ⟶ Oats or protein

Microwave meals ⟶ Batch-cooked real food

Artificial sweets ⟶ Dates, berries, dark chocolate

These weren't punishments — they were upgrades.

My clarity wasn't a miracle. It was the removal of fog.

What You Feed, Grows

Your brain is part of your body. And your body is affected by everything you put in it.

If you feed it junk, expect fog.

If you feed it clarity, expect change.

And when you experience that change — really feel it — you'll realise:

"The fog we call normal only clears when we stop feeding it."

Key Takeaway:

Most of what we call "normal" is actually just common. Real normal feels like clarity, energy, and peace.

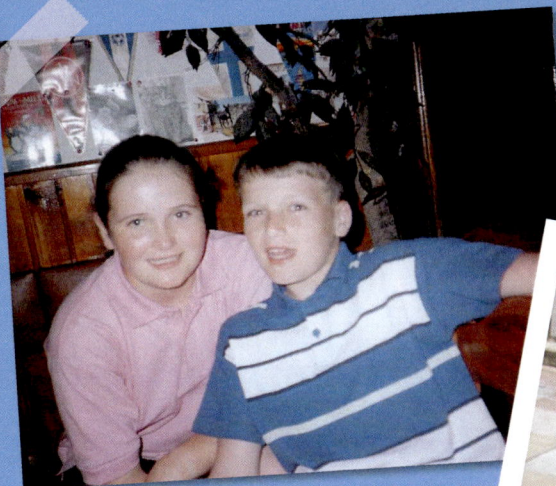
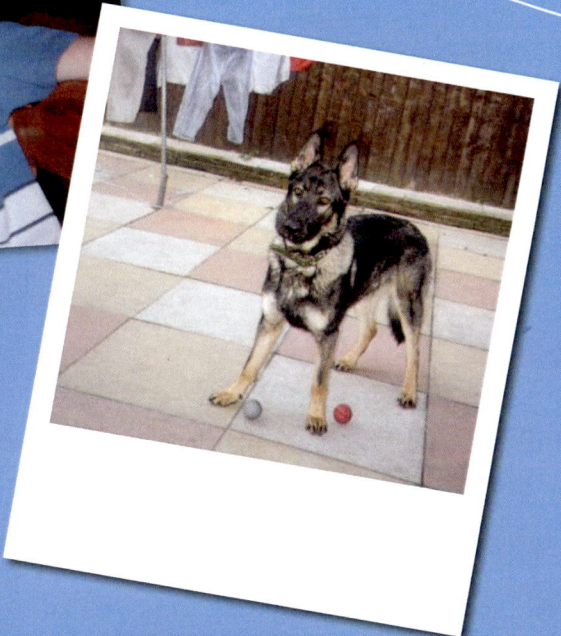
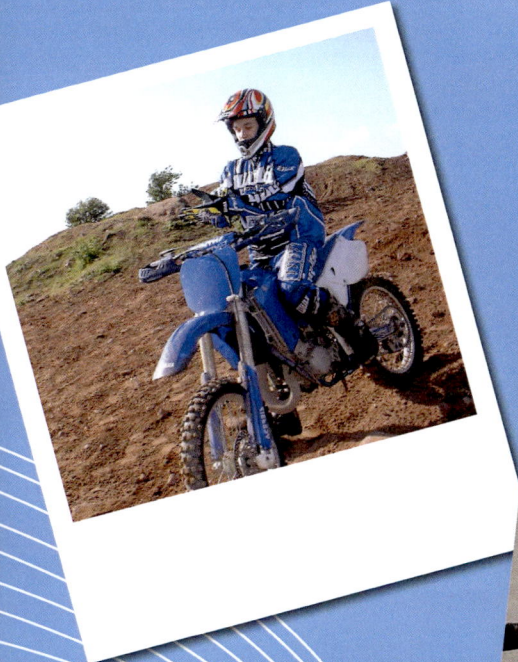
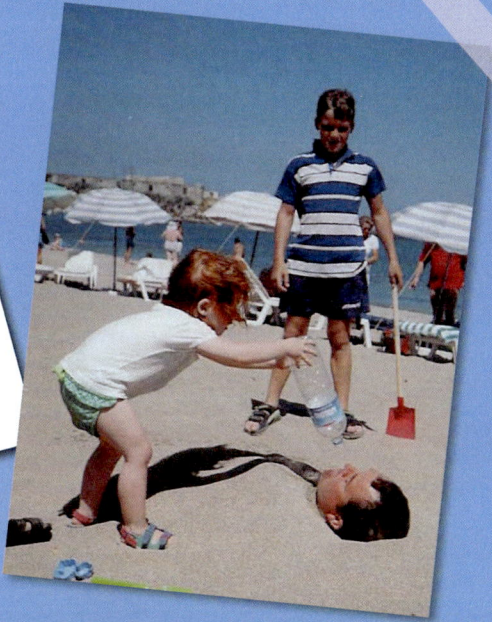

Chapter 3 - Part 1

Hidden in Plain Sight

We don't just eat food anymore.

We eat branding.

We eat marketing.

We eat convenience wrapped in lies.

The fog doesn't just come from what's in our food — it comes from what's sold to us as food.

If you've ever grabbed a "healthy" snack bar, a fruit drink, or a low-fat yoghurt thinking it was a smart choice — this chapter is for you.

Because the truth is: You've been tricked.

And it's not your fault.

The Illusion of Choice

Picture it: You walk into a supermarket to grab something "healthy."

You head for the "Good for You" aisle. Green labels. Slim fonts. Phrases like:

"No added sugar!"

"Low fat!"

"Made with real fruit!"

But flip the pack and what do you see?

Artificial sweeteners. Preservatives. E-numbers. Vegetable oil. Synthetic colours. Lab-made flavourings.

You weren't being offered choices.

You were being guided — manipulated — toward products designed to look healthy but deliver the same chemical fog.

Marketing vs. Reality

Here's what they say:

"Low fat" — Sounds good. But often means high sugar, fillers, and chemicals to make it taste like food again.

"All natural" — Legally meaningless. Even MSG (Monosodium Glutamate) can be called "natural."

"No added sugar" Usually means artificial sweeteners instead (like sucralose or aspartame).

"Gluten-free" — Helpful for some, yes. But doesn't make processed food healthy.

If it has to scream "I'm healthy!" on the front — it probably isn't.

Chapter 3 - Part 2

The Psychology of Packaging

Companies spend millions testing how colours, shapes, and words affect your decisions.

Yellow and red = trigger appetite (hello, fast food chains).

Green = signals health and eco.

Slim font = looks "cleaner" and lighter.

"Burst" graphics = urgency, fake freshness.

This is food design, not food nutrition.

And when you're neurodivergent — especially ADHD — you're even more susceptible to this kind of marketing manipulation. The brain seeks dopamine. Colourful packs, bold claims, and the promise of energy or focus hits that button.

The Additive Trap

Many of these "smart" food swaps contain a familiar list of hidden ingredients:

Maltodextrin – spikes blood sugar faster than glucose.

MSG (E621) – flavour enhancer linked to headaches and excitability.

Carrageenan – found in plant milks, can inflame the gut.

Artificial dyes – such as E133 or E102 - are still permitted in the UK, but banned in parts of Europe.

Even foods labelled as "diet," "light," or "high-protein" can be full of these.

It's hidden in plain sight — and legal.

The ADHD Amplifier

You might've grown up being called lazy, moody, or intense.

But imagine if your brain was never meant to be this foggy.

Imagine if food were pressing the wrong buttons.

Sugar highs.

Additive crashes.

Mood swings are tied to lunch.

Now layer ADHD on top — a brain already navigating dopamine dips, emotional regulation, sensory overwhelm…

No wonder so many of us feel broken.

My Wake-Up Moment

I remember one day, rushing into a shop between work estimates. I grabbed a "high-protein" wrap, an "immune-boosting" smoothie, and a sugar-free energy drink. Seemed like a sensible pick-me-up.

An hour later?

Heart racing.

Brain fog.

Mood tanked.

It wasn't the day.

It wasn't my job.

It was what I fed my brain.

So, I began scanning every label. I started seeing it everywhere — fake fibre, fake fruit, fake protein.

The fog wasn't just in my mind.

It was in the barcodes.

Take Back the Label

If you learn just one thing from this chapter, let it be this:

"The front of the pack is marketing. The back of the pack is the truth."

Start reading ingredients.

If it reads like a science experiment — leave it.

Real food doesn't need a bio.

An apple doesn't brag about being gluten-free.

Oats don't have a colourful banner saying "slow energy release."

You don't need to be perfect.

You just need to notice.

And from there, you unbox.

Key Takeaway:

Marketing sells stories. Ingredients tell the truth. Learn to read the back of the pack.

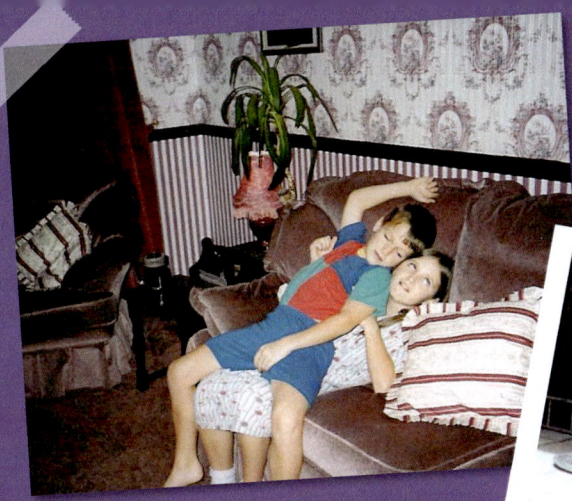

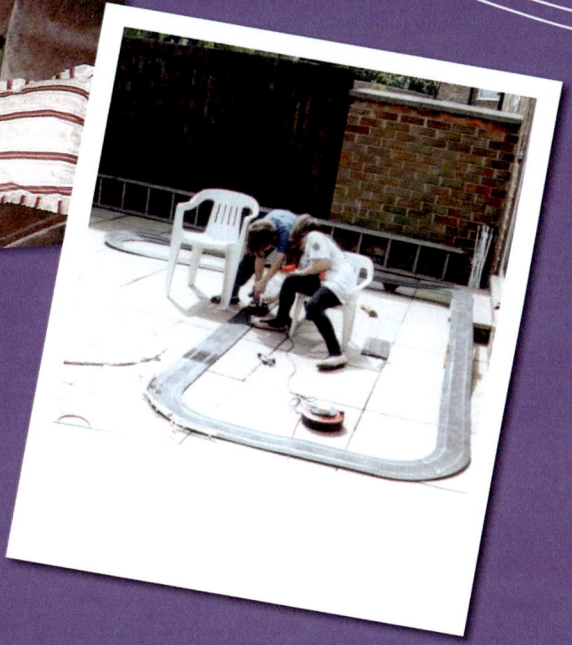

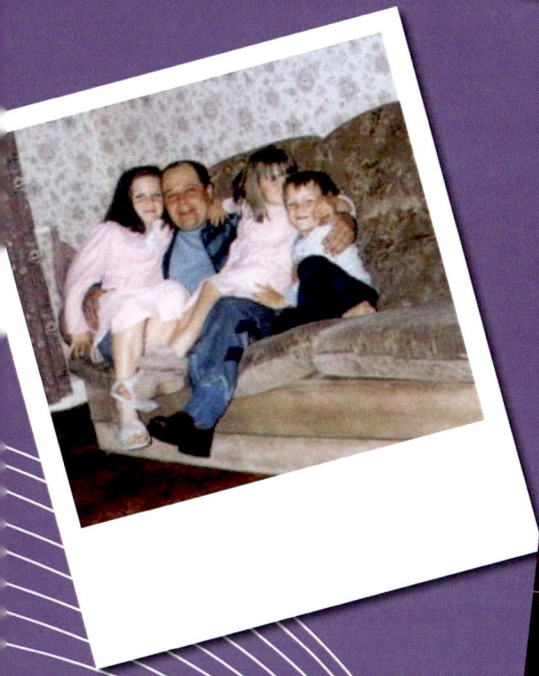

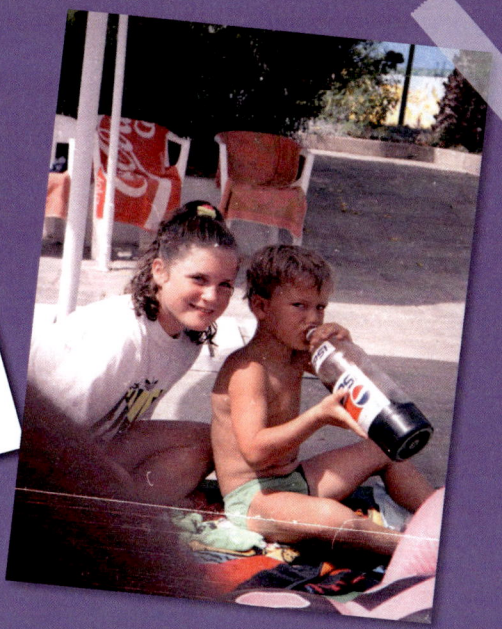

Chapter 4 - Part 1

Mood, Focus & Fog

We often think of our emotions and focus as things we have to wrestle with — discipline, motivation, and mindset. But what if a huge part of that struggle isn't mental at all?

What if it's chemical?

When You Can't Trust Your Own Mood

There was a time when I thought I was just moody. Or lazy. Or a bit short-tempered. Sometimes snappy, sometimes distant. I blamed myself, or the people around me, or life's constant stress.

But over time — and especially since cleaning up what I consumed — I started to see something else. Something sneaky. My moods weren't random. My energy didn't just dip. My focus wasn't unreliable "because I'm just like this."

It was food. It was chemicals. It was the crap I was putting into my body every single day, disguised as "normal."

The fog I thought was part of me was actually surrounding me.

And it wasn't until I stepped out of it that I realised how dense it had been.

Patterns That Weren't Personality

I remember one afternoon when I completely lost my rag over something small — some mess the kids had made, nothing major. I snapped, raised my voice, felt myself spiral. It wasn't until hours later that I realised I'd skipped breakfast, had two coffees and a handful of biscuits.

That wasn't me. That was a blood sugar spike and crash, caffeine overload, and no real nutrition.

It made me realise how often we punish ourselves for behaviours we never chose. How many parents beat themselves up for being short-tempered, or zoning out, or not having the energy to play, when the real issue might be the £1.20 energy drink and processed lunch they grabbed between errands.

Our inputs shape our outputs.

And we're not being told the truth about what we're taking in.

Chapter 4 - Part 2

The Misdiagnosed Fog

There's a version of fog that's so common, it's become invisible.

- You forget what you walked into a room for
- You start jobs but leave them unfinished
- You scroll your phone for hours and feel even worse after
- You lose your temper, then feel guilty, then numb
- You feel tired all the time

Doctors often call it stress, anxiety, or even depression. And sometimes, yes, it is.

But sometimes?

It's an allergic reaction. Or a sensitivity. Or a sugar crash. Or a hormonal disruption caused by additives you never realised you were eating.

I'm not saying food is the only answer. But if your body is under constant chemical attack, how can your brain possibly be clear?

My 72-Hour Clarity Rule

I started to notice something huge during my food experiments:

It took three days to feel clear.

Three days without additives. Three days with clean meals, early nights, and water.

Then the light would come back on.

It was like someone had lifted the blanket off my head. My thoughts became linear again. My patience returned. The noise in my mind dialled down. I could sit still, or get up and move, without a mental war first.

That's when I realised: So many of us think we're broken, when really, we're just fogged.

Check Your Inputs Before You Blame Your Outputs

Here are just a few things I realised were triggering mood swings or brain fog:

- Caffeine on an empty stomach
- Artificial sweeteners (especially aspartame and sucralose)
- Skipping meals, then binging carbs
- Multicoloured sweets or drinks (hello E-numbers)
- Lack of protein at breakfast
- Staying up past midnight scrolling

You don't need to overhaul your life overnight. But check your inputs.

Because when you're tired, overwhelmed, and unfocused — it might not be your fault. It might be your fuel.

You Are Not the Fog

This chapter isn't about guilt. It's about hope.

You don't need to become a food scientist or a Zen monk. You just need to pause. Notice. Swap what you can. Watch for patterns.

Because once you realise the fog isn't you, you can start clearing it.

And on the other side?

That's where you meet the version of yourself you were always meant to be.

Key Takeaway:

Your mood isn't your personality. Your focus isn't your character. Sometimes, it's just your fuel.

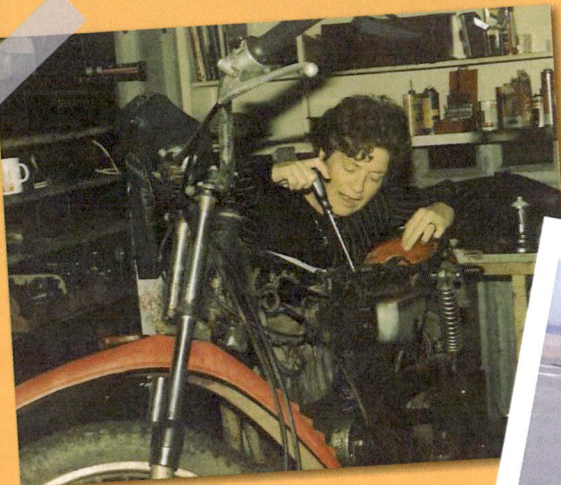
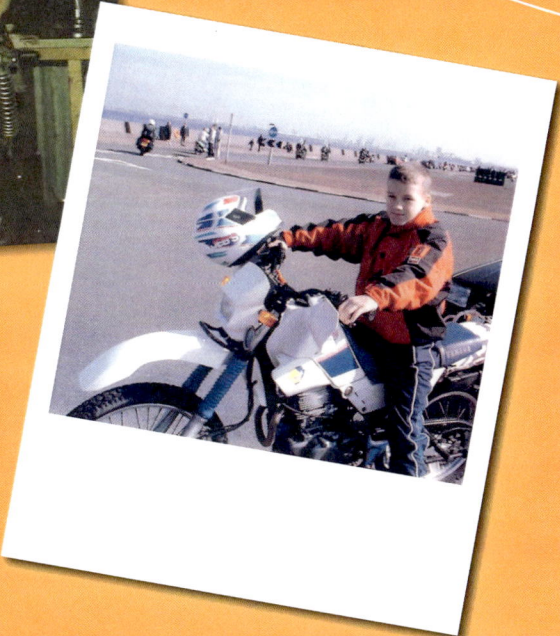
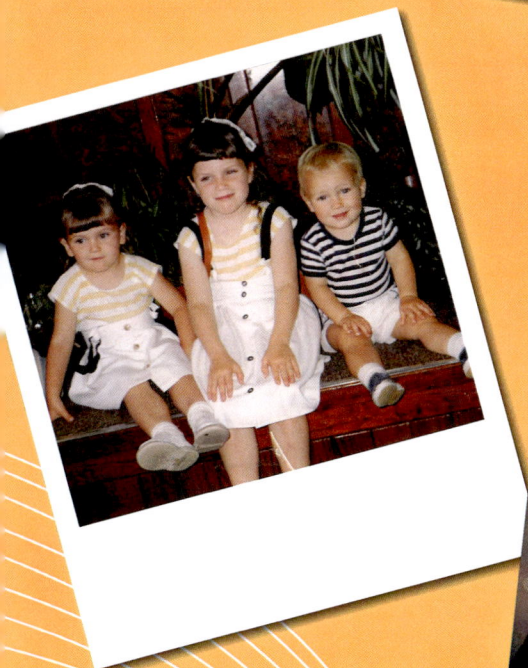
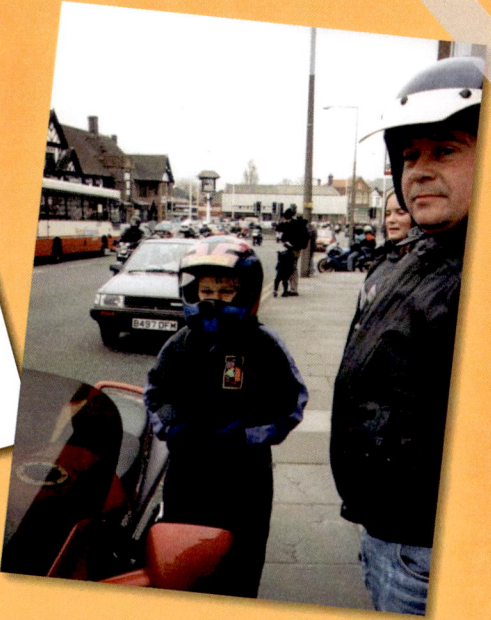

Chapter 5 - Part 1

The ADHD Connection

Most of my life, I thought I was just intense.

Too fast. Too deep. Too distracted. Too everything.

It wasn't until my diagnosis that I realised I wasn't broken — I was built differently.

And it wasn't until I changed my diet that I realised just how much that difference could be supported… or sabotaged.

A Brain Wired to Notice Everything

People with ADHD don't just "struggle to focus."

We notice everything. Every sound. Every flicker of light. Every thought that spins off into another one. Every possible outcome of a single conversation.

It's like living with twenty tabs open in your brain — and five are playing music you didn't ask for.

When you add food chemicals, artificial stimulants, and energy crashes into that mix, it's no wonder so many of us feel burnt out or emotionally volatile.

The Diet–Dopamine Loop

ADHD brains crave dopamine — the brain's reward chemical.

We often reach for:

- Sugar (quick energy + dopamine hit)
- Caffeine (stimulation + alertness)
- Junk food (comfort + texture)
- Scrolling (novelty + distraction)

But here's the trap:

These things give us a short-term boost and a long-term crash. And every crash increases the craving.

I was living on that loop.

I didn't know how much my habits were making my ADHD symptoms worse until I changed them.

What Helped Me Most

Here's what made the biggest difference:

• High-protein breakfasts (eggs, nuts, oats)
• Hydration before caffeine
• Removing artificial colours and preservatives
• Eating before long tasks
• Magnesium, Omega-3s, and Zinc
• Tracking my mood vs. food for 14 days

This wasn't about "fixing" my ADHD.

It was about finally supporting my brain.

Chapter 5 - Part 2

Seeing the Real Me

Once the fog lifted, I could see my strengths clearly:

- My pattern recognition
- My emotional depth
- My creative problem-solving
- My unstoppable hyperfocus when aligned with purpose

I stopped trying to be like everyone else — and started designing a life that worked for me, not against me.

If You've Ever Been Called Too Much...

Too sensitive. Too messy. Too hyper. Too spacey.

Maybe it's not that you're too much.

Maybe it's that you were never supported in the way you needed.

This chapter is a reminder:

ADHD isn't a flaw to fix. It's a brain to understand.

And when we feed that brain the right way — without the fog, without the shame — we finally get to see what's underneath.

It's not chaos. It's brilliance.

Waiting to be unboxed.

Living With the Volume Turned Up

I always felt like my mind had 20 tabs open — and I was trying to answer emails while a band played in the background, someone asked me deep life questions, and the fire alarm kept going off.

But that was just a Tuesday.

For most of my life, I thought this was normal. That everyone's brain worked like this. That everyone walked into a room and scanned every sound, every corner, every possible risk or task. That everyone had that internal itch to solve things that weren't broken yet.

I didn't know it had a name.

I didn't know it came with a cost.

Missing the Signs
(Even When They Were Obvious)

I had always been smart — good at fixing, building, noticing patterns. But I couldn't sit still. I'd lose things constantly. My mind would race, my emotions would spike, and I'd have these huge bursts of energy... followed by crashes.

Still, I got by.

I worked hard. I showed up. I masked it all.

But inside, I was drowning in noise. And because I'd always been able to "function," no one ever asked if I was struggling.

Not even me.

ADHD is like that.

Especially in adults.

Especially in men who are trying to hold everything together.

Especially when you've learned how to mask it so well that even your closest friends think you're just "wired differently."

It wasn't until I hit my wall — mentally, emotionally, physically — that I finally looked underneath the surface.

That's when I got diagnosed.

And suddenly, all the scattered pieces of my past made sense.

Chapter 5 - Part 3

ADHD Isn't a Deficit — It's a Different Operating System

The name's misleading: Attention Deficit Hyperactivity Disorder.

It sounds like something's broken.

But the truth?

My brain wasn't short on attention.

It was flooded with it.

Too much attention to everything — the hum of the fridge, the tone in someone's voice, the flicker of a light, a memory from 10 years ago, a random idea about a business I might start someday, and oh — did I forget to call the bank?

It's like having a Ferrari brain with bicycle brakes.

And unless you understand how to work with it, you burn out the engine trying to make it behave like something it's not.

The problem isn't the speed or intensity.

It's the constant effort to fit in a world that expects you to function like everyone else.

But when you stop seeing it as a flaw, and start building around it — that's when things shift.

That's when the fog begins to clear.

Fuel and Fire Don't Mix

What I didn't realise — and what most people don't — is how much ADHD brains are affected by diet, environment, and hidden triggers.

I always thought my crashes were part of the condition.

Turns out, they were often chemical.

I was eating foods full of additives known to mess with dopamine and blood sugar — the very things my brain was struggling to regulate.

I was relying on energy drinks, skipping proper meals, and taking medications full of dyes and fillers.

And wondering why I felt worse.

When I finally started cleaning up what I was eating — when I began tracking how certain foods and ingredients affected my focus, my mood, my energy — it was like flicking the lights on in a dark room.

It wasn't perfect.

But it was powerful.

Living With ADHD Isn't Just a Diagnosis — It's a Lens

Since the diagnosis, I've learned how to live differently.

I plan tasks in sprints, not marathons.

I use whiteboards, alarms, sticky notes — not to over-organise, but to externalise the chaos.

I stopped judging myself for needing structure.

I gave myself permission to rest before I crash.

I'm still impulsive sometimes. Still forget things.

But I also have a brain that solves problems before others even see them.

That connects dots most people miss.

That can hyperfocus for hours when it matters.

And now, I know how to feed it.

I know when I'm slipping.

And I know that "clarity" isn't just a lucky day — it's something I can build.

Chapter 5 - Part 4

You Might Not Have ADHD — But This Still Applies

Maybe you're not diagnosed.

Maybe you've never thought about it.

But here's something important:

The same additives, chemicals, and lifestyle traps that fog up ADHD brains affect everyone.

They just show up differently.

Brain fog, low mood, fatigue, forgetfulness — these aren't "normal," even if they're common.

And if your brain's been quietly screaming for help, there's a good chance it's been drowned out by what you've been feeding it.

That's what this chapter is for.

To say:

You're not lazy.

You're not broken.

You're not alone.

You just might be running a Formula 1 engine on diesel and wondering why it keeps stalling.

Key Takeaway:

"ADHD isn't just a condition. It's a clue. And when you follow it, you don't just treat a disorder. You uncover a path."

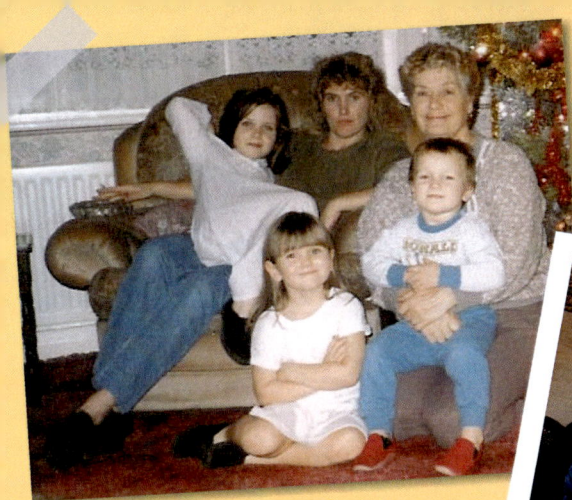
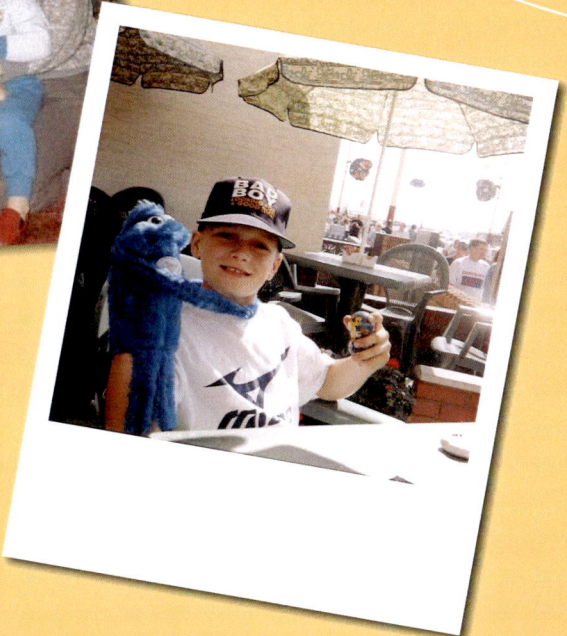
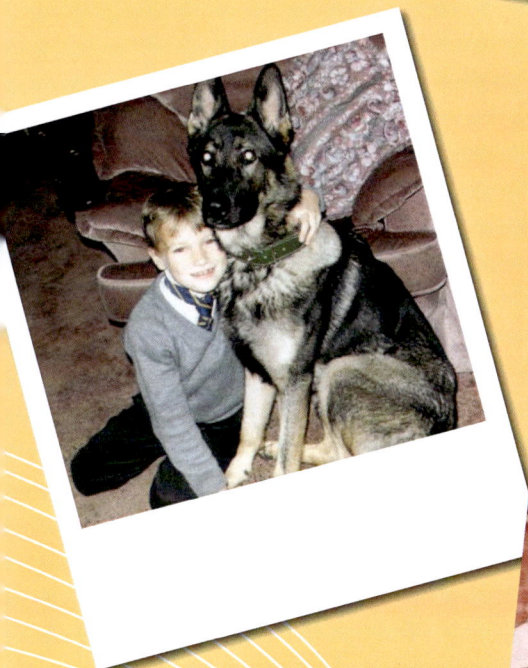
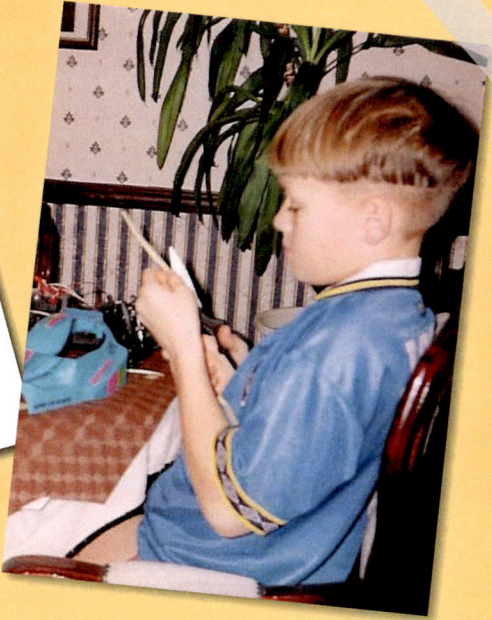

Chapter 6 - Part 1

Feeding the Fire

We don't just fall into the fog. We're led there.

No one wakes up craving E-numbers, aspartame, or beige freezer meals. We learn it. We're taught it. We're sold it. And once it's in our system long enough, we crave it — and feel worse without it.

When I look back now, it's almost comical. The foods I used to see as 'normal' were actually keeping me stuck. Not because I was lazy. Not because I had no willpower. **But because I was being baited every step of the way by products designed to hijack my brain, my focus, and even my mood.**

We think of addiction as a moral failing — something reserved for illegal substances. But what if the real addiction is packaged in colourful wrappers and pushed on us since birth?

Designed to Hook You

Walk down any supermarket aisle, and what do you see? Bright boxes. Buzzwords like "natural," "low fat," or "boosts immunity." Cartoons on cereal. Protein claims on chocolate bars. But flip the box around and you'll find a cocktail of preservatives, colourings, artificial sweeteners, and lab-made flavour enhancers. Even 'healthy' foods aren't always safe.

As someone with ADHD, I learned that my brain was more sensitive to dopamine swings — and these foods were engineered to exploit that sensitivity. The sugar hits, the caffeine bursts, the artificial flavour highs — all followed by the inevitable crash. I'd blame myself for not having energy or motivation when, really, my body was screaming for real fuel.

It's Not Just Food

It's your entire environment. The screens. The scrolling. The chaotic noise of modern life. Notifications. News. Noise. It all creates the same stimulation–crash cycle. Over time, you start to mistake stimulation for satisfaction. But they're not the same.

We're taught to chase quick hits — sugar, likes, caffeine, validation — and ignore the quiet work of healing. But real clarity isn't loud. It's steady.

Chapter 6 - Part 2

The System Is Set Up This Way

Let's not pretend this is random. There's an entire ecosystem profiting from your fog:

Food companies profiting from cheap, addictive fillers

Pharma companies sell pills for the symptoms

Marketing agencies make junk feel like joy

And people like us — neurodivergent, sensitive, emotionally intense — we're more vulnerable to it. More likely to be dismissed as anxious, moody, or lazy when really, we're burnt out from carrying what the world won't see.

I didn't want to believe that the world was set up this way. But once you see it, you can't unsee it.

My Own Fire

At my lowest, I wasn't just tired. I was wired and tired. Jumpy, foggy, distracted, emotionally flatlined. Then I'd get these bursts of motivation — hyperfocus, late-night rabbit holes, new business ideas — only to burn out a few days later. I thought it was just ADHD. But really, it was my lifestyle pouring petrol on it.

I was eating beige, thinking grey, living in static. And I couldn't understand why nothing changed.

Until I stepped back.

Until I Unboxed.

The Shift: What Real Fuel Looks Like

Swapping cereal for eggs. Water instead of energy drinks. Fresh food instead of frozen beige. It wasn't instant — nothing magic ever is — but within weeks, I noticed:

My mornings didn't feel like a fight

My mood wasn't bouncing all over the place

I could listen longer. Focus deeper. Rest better.

That's when it hit me: The fire I'd been feeding was burning me out —

but the right fuel could light me up.

Closing Message: You're Not Broken

If you're exhausted all the time, forgetful, snappy, distracted, hungry right after eating, or just numb — it doesn't mean you're broken.

It might just mean you're feeding the wrong fire.

Let's change what we fuel.

Key Takeaway:

What you feed grows. Feed the fog, get more fog. Feed clarity, get more clarity.

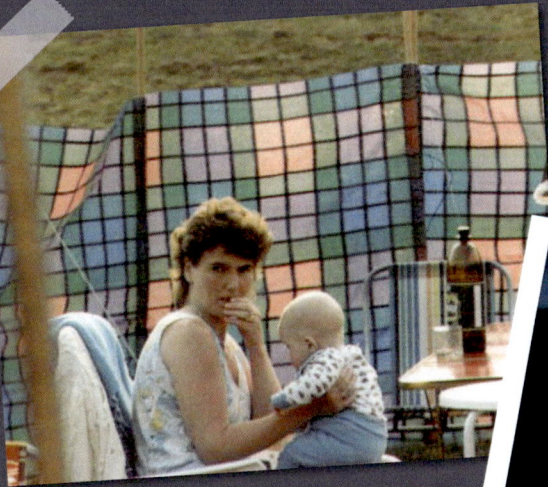
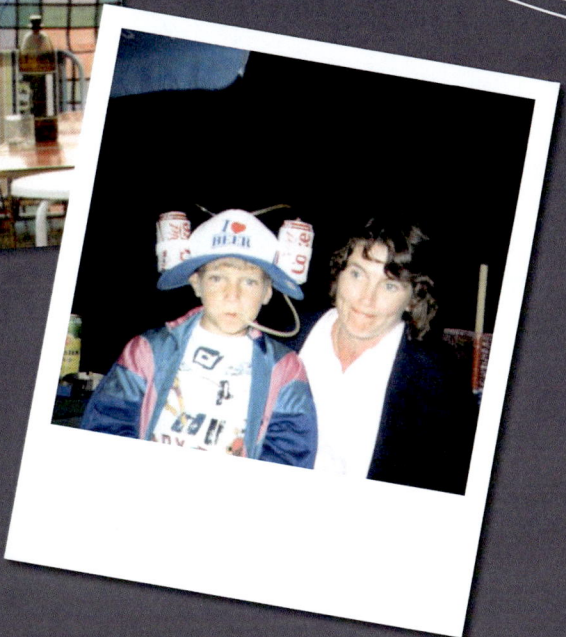
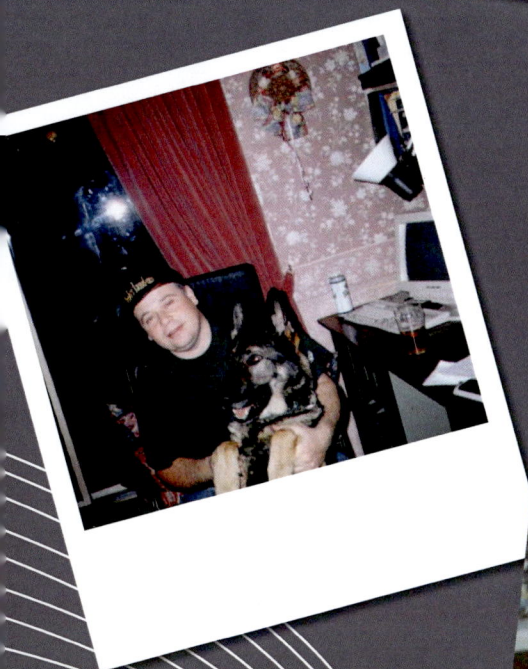
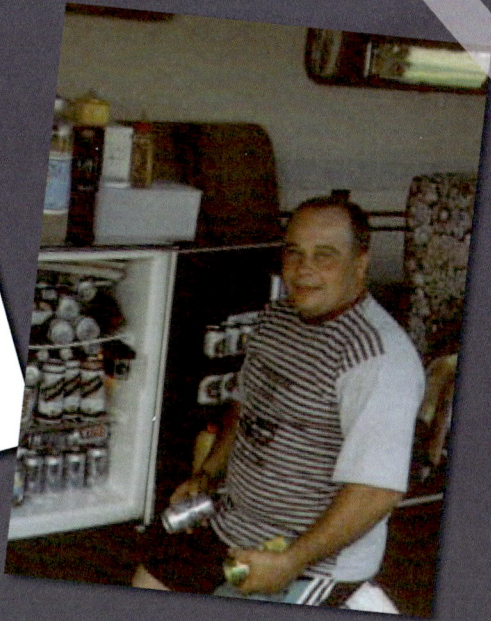

Chapter 7 - Part 1

Survival Mode

Why can't I stop eating this?

You ask yourself — mid-bite, mid-scroll, mid-stare into the fridge.

You're not hungry. You're not even enjoying it anymore.

But you keep going. And afterwards, you feel worse.

Then it begins…

The shame.

The "What's wrong with me?"

The "I'll start again Monday."

The promise you might keep.

But what if it's not your willpower that's broken?

What if it's your biology — hijacked?

Hooked By Design

Modern processed food is engineered to override your natural stop signals.

Your body evolved to crave:

Sugar (for quick energy)

Fat (for storage)

Salt (for hydration and preservation)

Now imagine combining those three — sugar, fat, and salt — with artificial flavourings, textures, crunch, colours, preservatives, excitotoxins, and clever packaging.

That's not food anymore.

It's a product.

A product tested and refined in labs to do one thing:

Keep you coming back.

And it works. Especially if you're tired, distracted, neurodivergent, or emotionally worn out.

Which, let's be honest, most of us are.

The ADHD Factor

If your brain already struggles with impulse control, delayed gratification, or dopamine regulation…

You're the perfect customer.

The same brain that helps you hyperfocus, imagine wildly, or feel deeply is also the brain that feels urgent relief when you crack a can of cola or rip open a shiny wrapper.

Dopamine hits. Temporarily.

And that's not weakness — it's wiring.

Processed foods target the same reward systems as drugs, gambling, or social media.

Only difference?

They're sold on every corner.

Legal. Cheap. Socially accepted.

Even encouraged.

"Treat yourself."

"You deserve it."

"Go on, one won't hurt."

Chapter 7 - Part 2

When Fuel Becomes Filler

There's a point where food stops being fuel and starts being filler.

Filler for:

Stress

Boredom

Loneliness

Exhaustion

Emotional gaps we haven't even named yet

And because those gaps don't get filled, we keep reaching.

You're not addicted to biscuits.

You're looking for clarity, comfort, and connection.

And you've been sold a shortcut that doesn't work.

The Sugar-Stress Spiral

This one's especially sneaky:

You're stressed

You reach for sugar

Sugar spikes insulin

Insulin crashes your blood sugar

Your mood drops

You feel more stressed

So… you reach again

A cycle.

Wearing your body down.

Training your nervous system to expect instant relief, instead of real restoration.

CHAPTER 7 - PART 2

Over time, this blunts your ability to feel "normal" without a crutch.

And that becomes your baseline.

Your new fog.

Unboxing the Craving

Here's what helped me break the cycle:

1. Pause before you reach

Ask: What am I actually feeling right now?

2. Swap just one thing

Not everything. One.

(Fruit instead of sweets. A walk instead of a scroll.)

3. Pre-load good food

Don't wait to be starving. Start with what fuels.

4. Don't go to war with yourself

You're not lazy. You're overridden.

That's different — and fixable.

5. Sleep, light, hydration

It's not all food. It's how you live between meals, too.

This Is Survival Brain

You're not greedy.

You're not broken.

You're surviving in a world that sells comfort instead of healing.

Your ancient instincts are being played by modern products.

But every time you pause…

Every time you notice…

Every time you choose real over fake…

You're rewiring survival back into strength.

You're Not Alone

Millions of people feel exactly like this.

Shame keeps it quiet.

But it's time to speak up.

We're not lazy.

We're exhausted.

We're fogged up by design.

And we're waking up.

Key Takeaway:
"Cravings don't make you weak. They're signals. Unbox them."

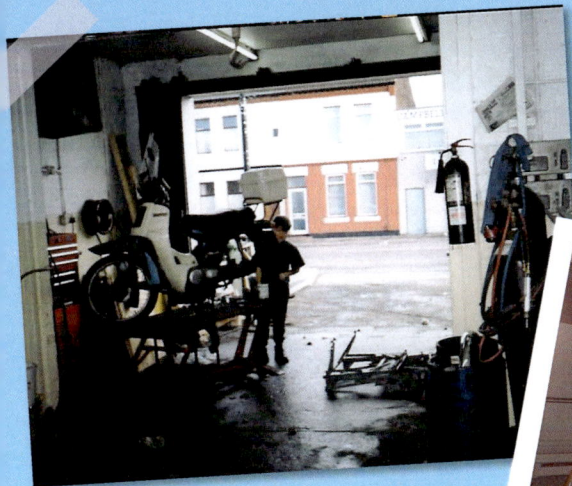
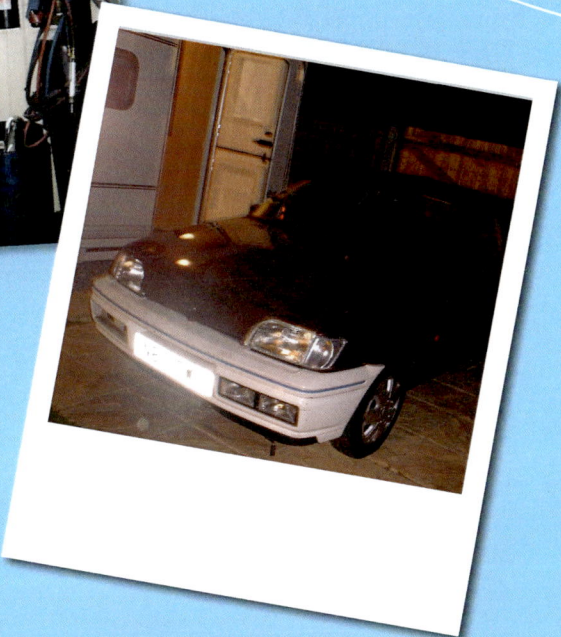
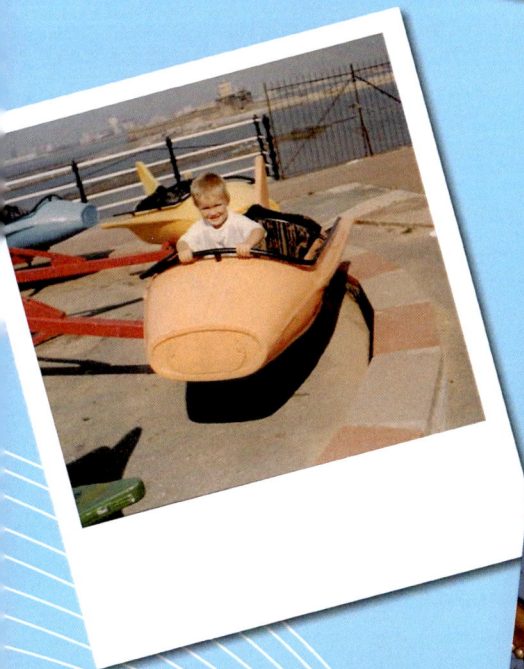
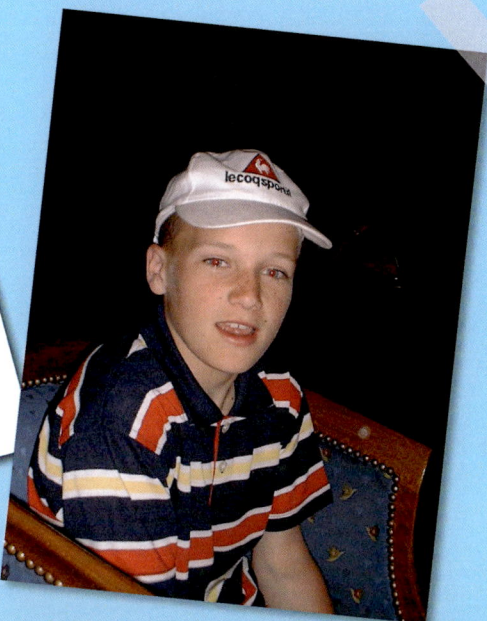

Chapter 8 - Part 1

Fuel vs. Food

What are we really feeding?

Most people think they're eating to fuel their bodies.

But when you zoom out, most modern diets aren't fuelling anything — they're just filling.

We eat for:

Comfort

Energy bursts

Social norms

Habit

And, let's be honest… marketing

But fuelling is different. Fuel is purposeful. It's measured. It supports performance, clarity, and growth.

Food — real food — is fuel.

Much of what we consume today, though, is simply engineered filler.

What Your Body Actually Needs

Your body is an engine.

But not one from the 1950s — this thing is Formula 1.

It needs:

Clean carbohydrates for energy

High-quality fats for hormones and brain health

Protein to repair and build

Hydration to regulate it all

Micronutrients (like magnesium, zinc, B-vitamins) to keep the wiring firing right

But now look at most supermarket trolleys.

We've replaced fuel with fillers:

Processed sugar for energy (followed by a crash)

Vegetable oils instead of essential fats

Caffeine to fake focus

Additives to make lifeless food addictive

Preservatives so that food can sit on shelves longer than a houseplant

And we wonder why our minds are wired, our bodies inflamed, and our energy unpredictable.

What Additives Feed

Every bite feeds something.

You either feed:

Focus or fatigue

Calm or chaos

Repair or inflammation

Clarity or confusion

Additives feed confusion. They overstimulate one system and suppress another.

Artificial sweeteners may spike insulin. Synthetic colours can disrupt mood. Preservatives tax the liver.

And when your body's detox systems are overwhelmed?

It stores the toxins in fat.

The body literally hides the damage just to keep you functioning.

But you feel it… in your fog. Your mood. Your motivation.

Chapter 8 - Part 2

Is Your Diet Fuelling the Problem?

Here's the thing I realised:

You can be eating plenty and still be starving — at a cellular level.

That's what was happening to me.

I'd have a full stomach… but zero mental energy.

I'd eat meals loaded with flavour… but still feel low.

Why?

Because what I was feeding wasn't me.

It was:

Cravings driven by additives

Emotional habits built during burnout

Marketing tricks telling me "This bar = health"

And food-like products, not food

The difference became crystal clear when I finally stripped it back.

Real food gave me real energy.

Not a fake high… but lasting, steady, calm energy.

Food That Fuels

Fuel-food isn't just about kale and quinoa.

It's about feeding your function.

Here's what I started leaning into:

Craving Type | Typical Fix | Fuel-Based Upgrade

Sweet | Sugary snacks | Dates, berries, raw honey

Crunchy | Crisps & crackers | Roasted chickpeas, seeds

Energy crash | Energy drinks | Water, electrolytes, fruit

Quick lunch | Sandwich meal deal | Eggs, veg, brown rice

Once I changed the intention from "eating to feel full"

To "eating to function well" …

Everything changed.

Marketing Makes the Confusion Worse

Walk through any "healthy" food aisle and you'll see:

Protein bars with more additives than a Mars bar

Cereal claiming to support heart health… while being 35% sugar

Low-fat yoghurt packed with stabilisers and colours

Gluten-free labels on food that never had gluten to begin with

That's the trick: It looks like food.

But it doesn't act like fuel.

Your body isn't fooled.

It just has to work harder to compensate.

Fuelling Focus, Mood & Motivation

Once I made the shift, here's what changed first:

Mornings: I didn't need caffeine just to feel alive.

Mood: I was less reactive. More stable.

Energy: Lasted beyond lunch. No more 2 pm crash.

Sleep: Came naturally — deep, unbroken.

Motivation: The fog lifted. The fire returned.

And I realised…

I'd been giving my body the wrong fuel for years and wondering why it didn't run properly.

Chapter 8 - Part 3

So... What Are You Feeding?

Are you feeding the part of you that wants peace, progress, presence?

Or the one that's running from stress, soothing pain, numbing out?

Food is more emotional than we realise.

It's tied to culture, trauma, and identity.

But it's also your body's main information source.

Every bite is a message.

The more real the food, the clearer the signal.

Unboxed Reflection

You don't need to overhaul your whole diet overnight.

Just start noticing.

What foods make you feel foggy?

Which ones bring clarity?

What are you feeding when you eat that thing?

Because what you feed grows.

Key Takeaway:

Food is information. What message are you sending your body?

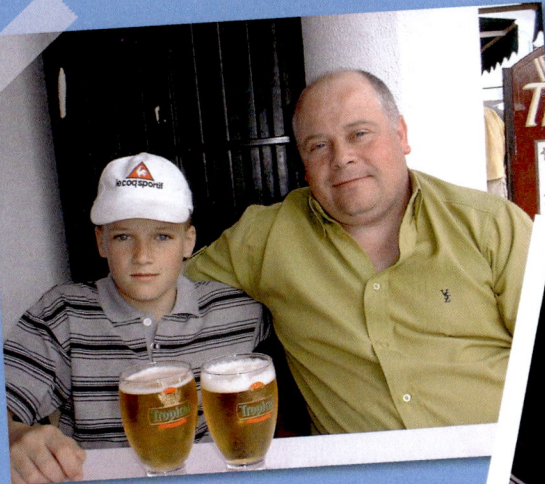
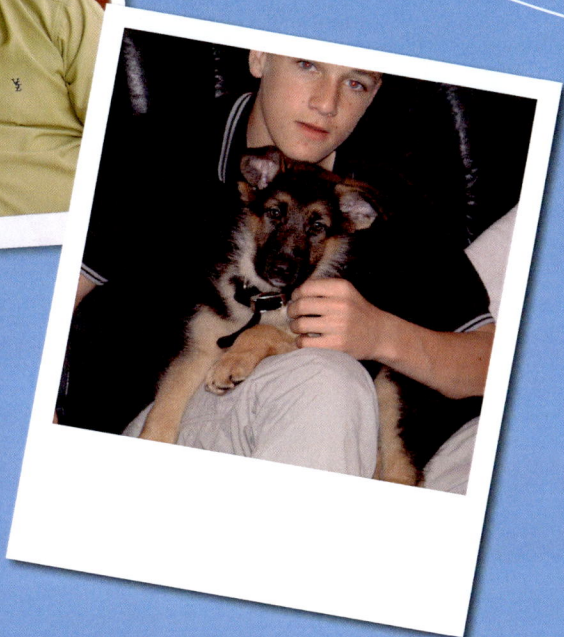
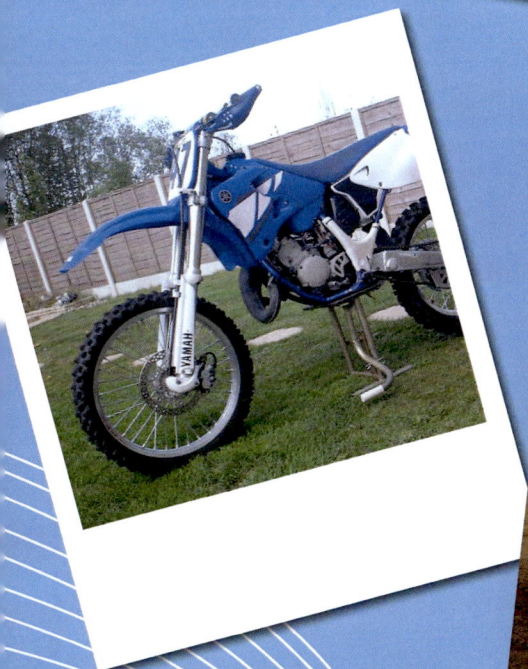
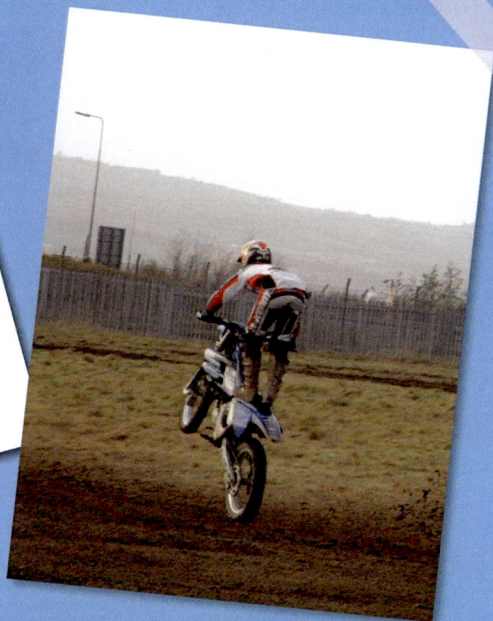

Chapter 9 - Part 1

Detoxing Body & Mind

We often imagine detoxing as a frantic rush to flush everything out — a weekend juice cleanse, a social media fast, a sweat-soaked gym session that promises redemption. But detoxing isn't a punishment. It's not about guilt. **It's about giving your body and brain space to breathe. Room to reset.** And when you've been running on processed chaos for years — emotionally and physically — detoxing becomes less of a health fad and more of a survival tool.

It's about clearing the fog, layer by layer.

The Layers That Trap Us

At first, you think it's just your energy that's low. Then you realise your thoughts aren't as clear. You forget things, you zone out mid-conversation, your moods swing without warning. You start snapping more. Or shutting down.

And here's the kicker — you think it's just you. **But what if it's what's in you?**

Your body keeps the receipts. Years of E-numbers, sweeteners, ultra-processed meals, energy drinks, medications, and even the chemicals in your shampoo — all compounding over time. For some, these additives get flushed easily. For others, especially those with ADHD, PCOS, or autoimmune issues, it builds up like traffic on a Friday night. Blocked. Fogged. Wired.

When I started noticing this, I couldn't unsee it. My skin looked different. My breath smelled different. I could taste chemicals hours after eating. I could feel the tension in my stomach. And weirdly, the more I stripped things back, the more the fog started to lift.

Step One: Simplify to See

Before you do anything radical, try this:

One day of eating only real food. No barcodes. No labels. No ingredient lists. Just fruit, veg, rice, eggs, meat or fish — things your nan would recognise.

One day of drinking only water, herbal tea, or proper homemade juice.

One day off the screens, if you can. Go for walks. Nap. Breathe.

You'll start to notice things almost immediately — not perfection, but signals: bloating shifts, your jaw unclenches, you're less irritable. That's your body talking. **Now imagine if it had seven days to speak.**

Chapter 9 - Part 2

Detox Is Not One Size Fits All

Everyone's baseline is different. Some people can smash energy drinks and sleep fine. Others can have one Diet Coke and feel wired for hours. This isn't about copying someone else's plan. **It's about experimenting.**

Create a log — or use the Unboxed app when it's live. Track:

How you feel before/after eating

What additives you had (we'll help you ID them)

Sleep, digestion, mood, and focus

You're not broken. You're just running a system that's overloaded. Detoxing is about lightening that load so your real self can start to r e-emerge.

Let's Talk About Vaping

Now here's something that rarely gets mentioned — especially in wellness circles trying to sell you crystals and kombucha.

Most vape liquids contain glycerol or propylene glycol. These are generally safe in small amounts — until you overheat them. When the coil burns too hot — either through poor maintenance, chain vaping, or "dry hits" — glycerol can break down into acrolein, formaldehyde, and acetaldehyde.

Acrolein is a known lung irritant.

Formaldehyde is a probable human carcinogen, used in embalming fluid.

Acetaldehyde is also linked to DNA damage.

We're not here to guilt-trip — but knowledge is power. If you're vaping, make sure your coil is clean, avoid dry hits, and take breaks. Some people might genuinely find it helps them avoid worse habits — but it's not risk-free.

We'll have harm-reduction tips in the Unboxed app too, because quitting cold turkey isn't realistic for everyone.

Real Detox Starts with Ownership

Detoxing isn't glamorous. It's messy, emotional, and sometimes lonely. You'll second-guess yourself. You'll get annoyed that you can't just eat what everyone else eats. But then, you'll feel yourself again.

You'll feel that little switch flip — the moment your brain fires clearer,

your body calms, and your old self whispers: "I've missed you."

That's detoxing Unboxed style. No extremes. No shame. Just you, stepping back into the driver's seat.

Next stop? Building a new lifestyle — one that doesn't need rescuing from.

Key Takeaway:

Detoxing isn't about punishment. It's about creating space for your real self to emerge.

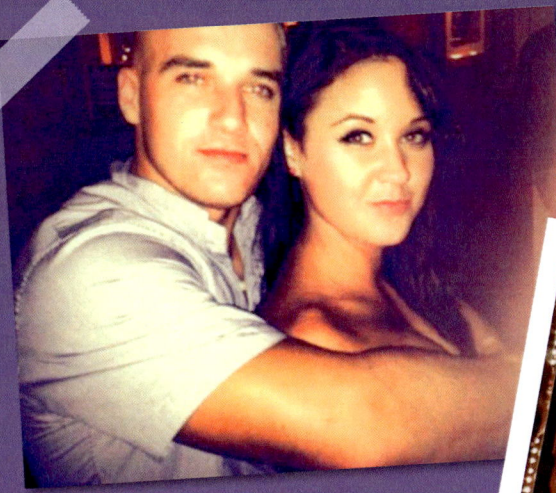
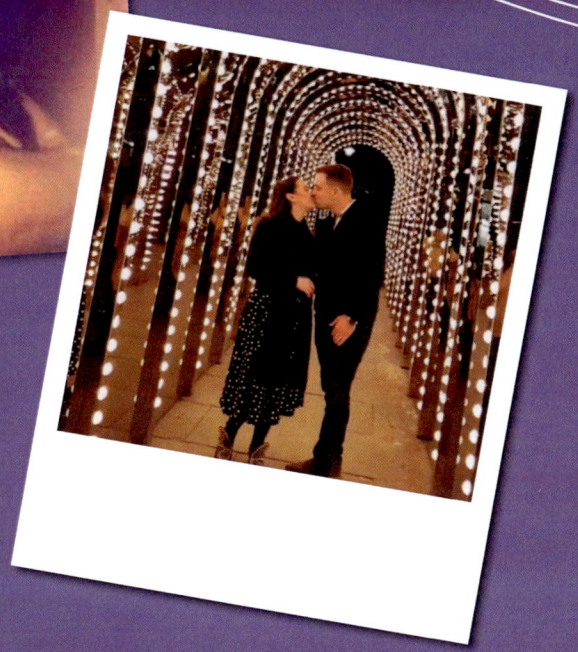
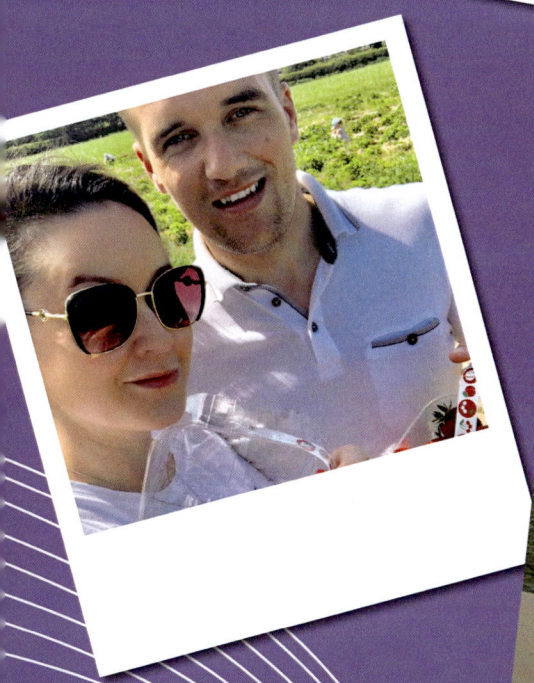
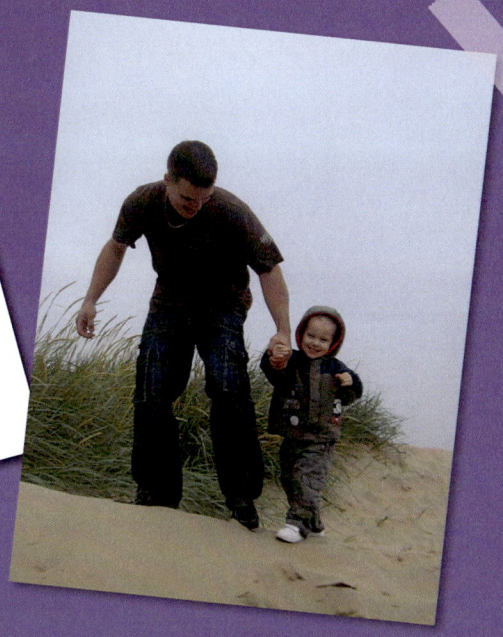

Chapter 10 - Part 1

Living Unboxed
The Return to Clarity

It's a strange feeling when the fog finally lifts.

You spend so long thinking it's just who you are — tired, snappy, unmotivated. That everything you didn't do yesterday is just more proof you're lazy, or broken, or just can't cope like others seem to.

But then something happens.

You realise: It wasn't you.

It was the chemicals, the chaos, the conditioning.

The invisible weight of a system built to keep you too distracted, too wired, or too exhausted to notice.

Wait... this is how I'm supposed to feel?

The first time I woke up with energy — real energy — I thought it was a fluke.

I hadn't changed much yet. But I had removed a few things:

– The fizzy drinks I thought were harmless

– The late-night snacks are full of additives

– The ultra-processed lunches I told myself were "fine in moderation"

And in return?

Clarity. Lightness. Calm.

It wasn't a buzz. It wasn't like caffeine or meds.

It was just... peace.

The kind of peace you don't even realise you've never had, until you feel it for the first time.

Small wins. Big shifts.

I didn't become some clean-eating monk overnight.

There were slip-ups. There still are.

But with each day of better choices, the "real me" became easier to reach.

I started noticing patterns:

When I ate well, my patience returned.

When I avoided certain additives, I didn't snap as quickly.

When I hydrated, I could think more clearly.

When I planned even simple meals, I felt in control again.

It wasn't about restriction. It was about reclaiming myself.

Chapter 10 - Part 2

Unboxing isn't a detox. It's a lifestyle.

There's no finish line. No magical "fully clean" state.

What there is — is awareness.

And once you see it, you can't unsee it.

You start to look at your cupboard differently.

You start to notice how you feel after you eat, not just how it tastes.

You begin to understand that every product is designed to win your attention, not your health.

And you stop giving your energy away so freely.

Clarity gives you a choice.

Once you clear the fog, you get to decide:

What kind of parent, partner, or friend do you want to be

What work do you put into the world

What rest looks like on your terms

What fuel supports your body — not fights against it

You're no longer reacting. You're responding.

And the best part?

You're not doing it for anyone else's approval.

You're doing it because you finally get to feel like you again.

You'll start inspiring people without trying.

When people see your eyes brighter...

When you stop saying "I'm just tired" all the time...

When you smile more, snap less, and show up more fully...

They'll notice.

They'll ask:

"What are you doing differently?"

And you'll smile.

Because you'll know —

You didn't join a diet.

You didn't find some secret pill.

You just started unboxing the truth.

Unboxed isn't a fix. It's a return.
To clarity. To calm.
To who you were always meant to be.

Key Takeaway:

Living Unboxed isn't about perfection. It's about awareness, choice, and returning to your true self.

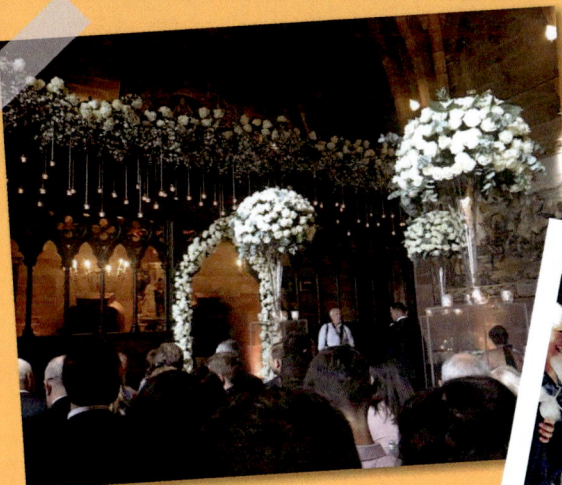

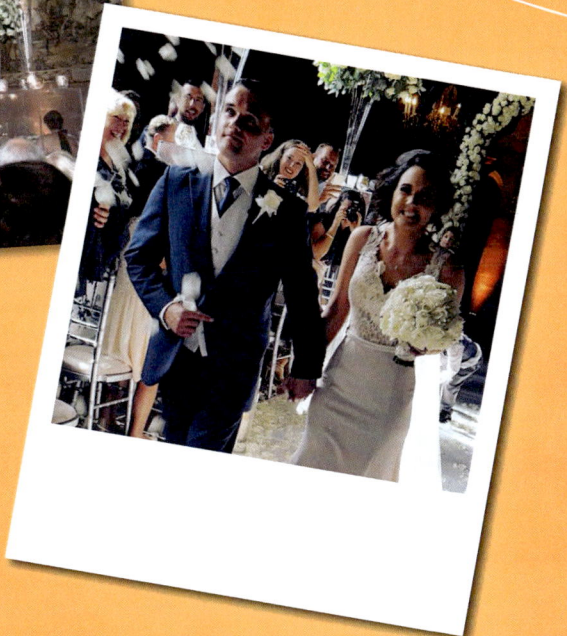

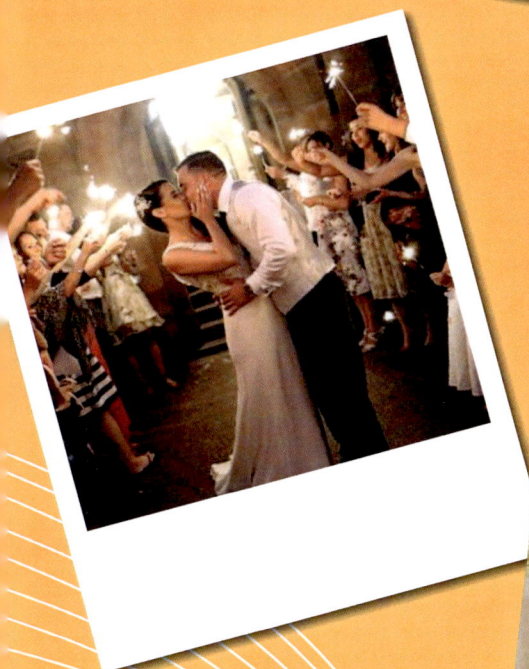

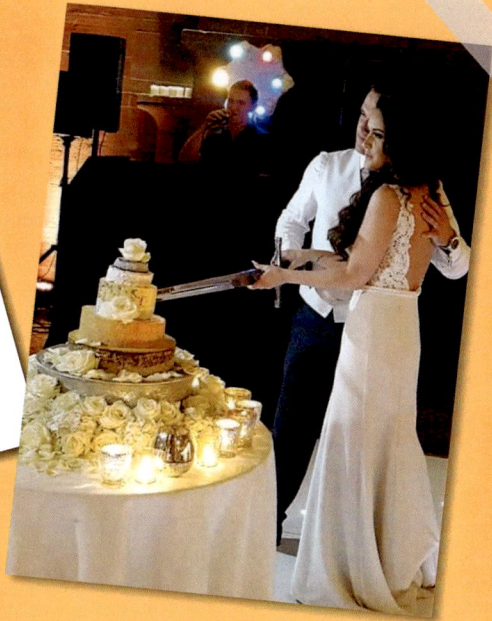

Chapter 11 - Part 1

The New You
Rewiring from the Roots Up

We spend most of our lives thinking change is about willpower. That if we just tried harder, we could stay off sugar, be more organised, less reactive, more present, sleep better, and feel clearer. But that version of "trying harder" doesn't work when you've been wired for chaos since childhood. It doesn't work when your system has been fogged up with junk, inside and out.

This isn't about turning into someone else.

This is about becoming more of who you actually are — once the interference is removed.

Burnout Wasn't My End — It Was My Upgrade Prompt

The worst part of my life didn't come from "doing nothing."

It came from trying to be everything.

To everyone.

It came from being switched on all the time, running on sugar, caffeine, nicotine, pushing through mental fog with a tired smile, doing DIY at midnight, checking invoices at 2 am, and doing a quote on my phone in the car before school drop off. I never paused long enough to ask if I was actually okay.

When the burnout came — the crash — I thought I'd failed. I thought I'd lost my edge. But it was the first time my body got a word in. The fog wasn't just in my mind. It was everywhere: in the food, in the stress, in the additives, in the pressure to never stop.

Once I accepted that, I realised...

I didn't need more willpower. I needed less noise.

Clarity Isn't a Buzzword — It's a State of Living

You know that feeling when your phone finally updates, and everything feels smooth again?

That was me — but as a person.

My thoughts used to trip over each other, like a dozen radios playing different stations at once. But now, they land one at a time. I still have ADHD. I still get ideas bouncing around. But I can choose what to tune into now. **That was never an option before.**

This new version of me is still fast-thinking, still passionate, still full of energy — but no longer burning out the circuits.

The power isn't gone.

It's finally directed.

Chapter 11 - Part 2

The Small Wins Are the Real Ones

People expect fireworks after the transformation. But in real life, it's more like:

Waking up without the tight chest.

Laughing more.

Being present with the kids, not just nearby.

Having energy left after work, not just collapsing.

You don't need to move to Bali or juice celery for 60 days.

You need to understand your wiring, your inputs, and your environment.

The real win?

When you can finally trust yourself again.

People Noticed — And Not Just Me

My mates, my kids, my wife — they all noticed it. Not just physically, but emotionally. I was less reactive, more thoughtful. I had patience I didn't even know I owned.

Clarity gave me back my kindness.

Even strangers started asking me what I'd changed.

At first, I didn't know how to explain it.

Now, I just say, "I stopped fogging up my brain."

Because it's true. And because I want them to know it's possible.

You Don't Have to Be Broken to Begin

I used to think you had to hit rock bottom to change. But you don't. **You just need one honest moment. One crack of light.**

That might be this chapter for you.

And if you have hit rock bottom? Then maybe, like me, you're about to meet the version of yourself that's been buried under the fog.

Not a better version.

Just a clearer one.

Key Takeaway:

The new you isn't someone different. It's you — without the interference.

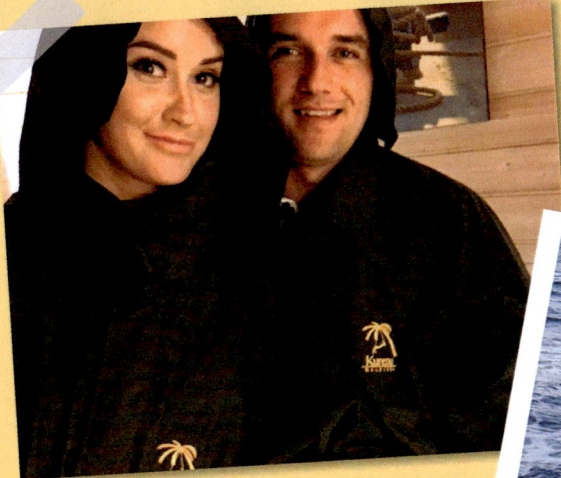
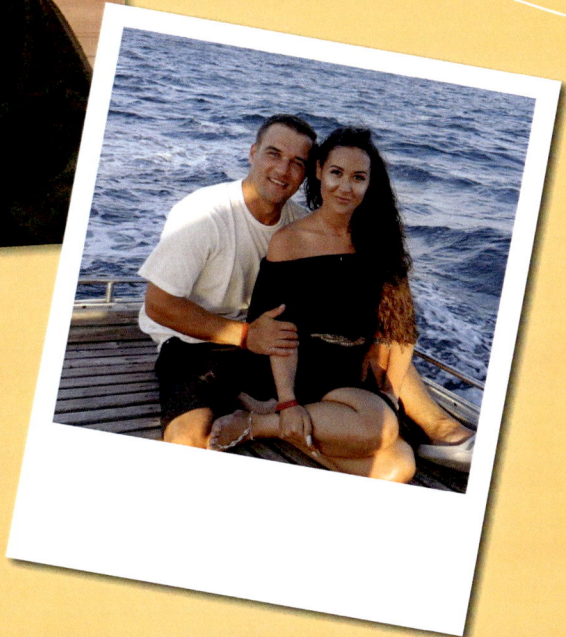
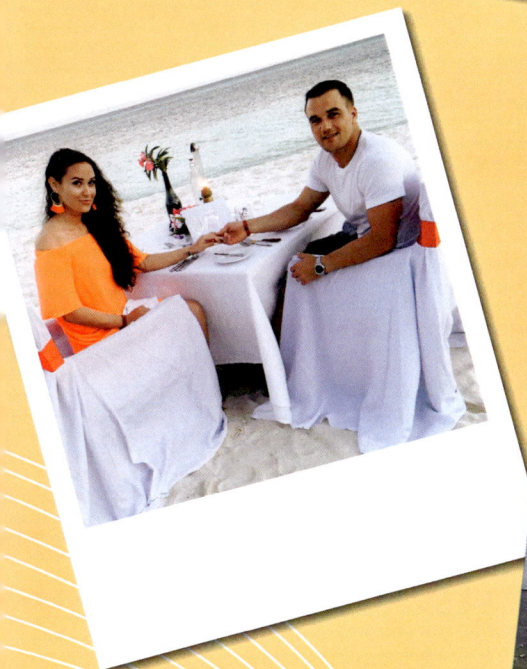
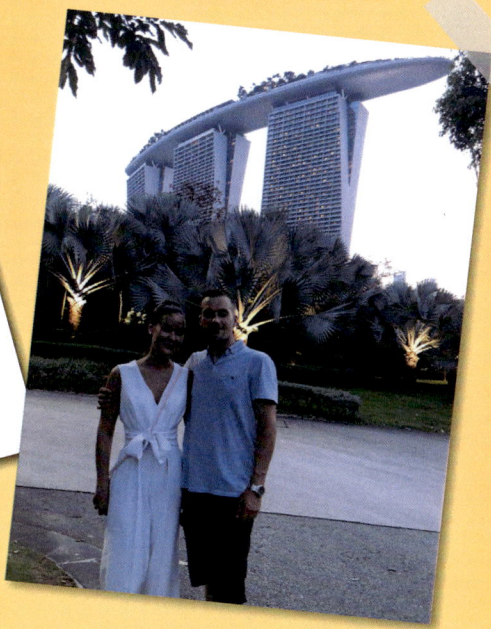

Chapter 12

Legacy & Community

Give One. Get One Donated. Build Something That Lasts.

What's the point of waking up — if you leave the rest of the world asleep?

Once I got my clarity back, that question started haunting me, not in a dark way, but in a purposeful one.

Because once you feel the fog lift — and you know how avoidable it really was — it becomes impossible to just walk past someone still stuck in it.

Especially when that someone looks like your past self.

This Isn't Just About Me Anymore

The start of this story was deeply personal: my fog, my health, my burnout, my healing.

But the destination?

It's about us.

It's about every parent who thinks exhaustion is just normal.

Every teen survives on energy drinks and dry cereal.

Every person who feels like they're constantly behind, wondering why life feels so heavy.

They deserve clarity, too.

But most of them won't get there with a £30 supplement or a 12-week plan.

They need something more real. More human.

And that's why Unboxed exists.

The Model: Give One, Get One Donated

When someone buys this book, they're not just buying it for themselves.

They're also donating one to someone who can't.

Someone on a waiting list for ADHD diagnosis.

A mum overwhelmed with life, looking for answers.

A man going through burnout who doesn't even have words for it yet.

A teen living on Monster and microwave meals, thinking that fog is just life.

One book. Two people helped.

Simple. Powerful. Fair.

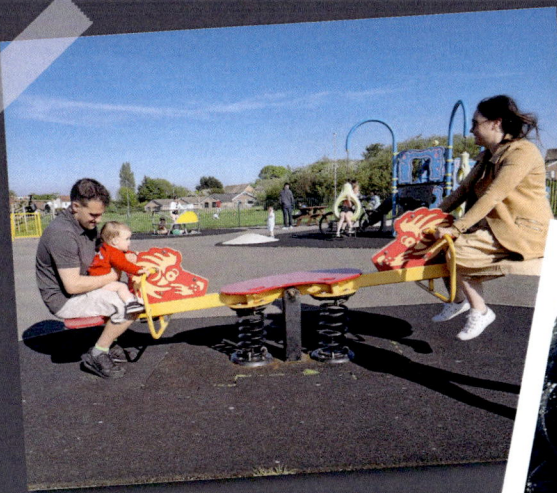

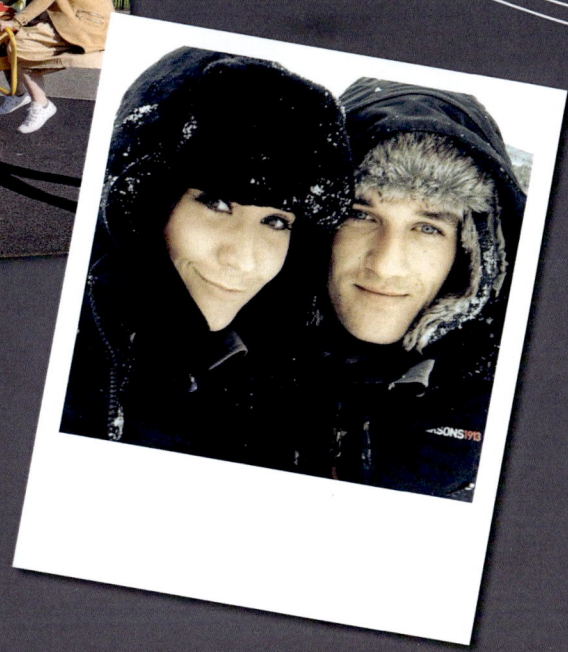

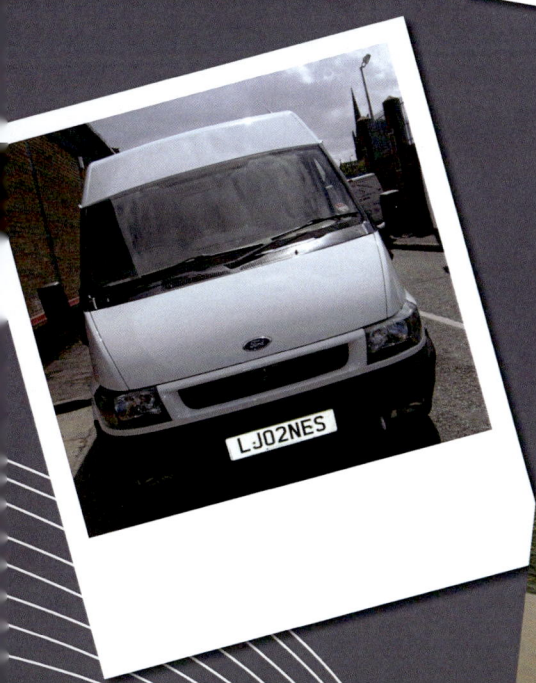

LJ02NES

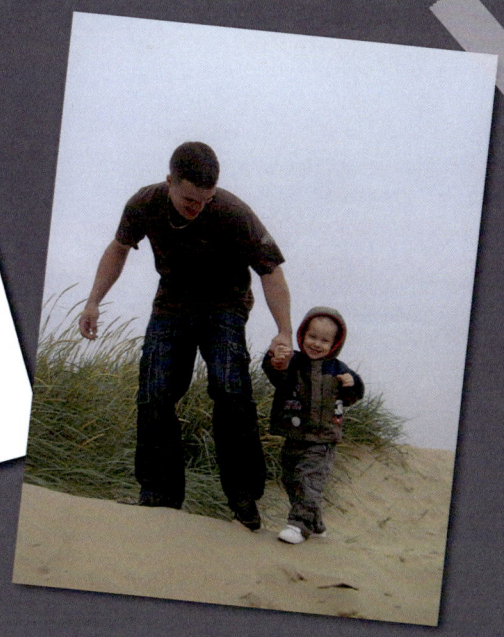

Chapter 13 - Part 1

Cannabis, Clarity & Coming Home to My Mind

There was a moment in Ibiza where everything stopped.

Not the world. Not time. Just the spinning, racing, tangled-up storm inside my head.

And in that pause — as quiet hit like a wave — I realised something terrifying:

I couldn't feel my own thoughts anymore.

Not clearly. Not like before.

They used to bounce with meaning. Pattern. Purpose.

Now they just buzzed. Loud. Broken. Blurry.

And that's when it hit me —

I used to feel like myself when cannabis was in the background.

I didn't even realise it at the time.

I wasn't "high." I wasn't "escaping."

I was clearing the fog — without knowing how thick it would become when I stopped.

At the time, quitting made sense. I was starting a family. Building a new life.

And for a while, I did feel better.

Or so I thought.

We had our first child. Life was bright.

Then came our second, just 15 months later. A beautiful daughter — my little Jen.

Two boys and now a tiny version of my wife. I was complete.

But so was the load.

Less sleep. More pressure. No time. No space.

And no silence in my mind.

What started as small cracks became deep fractures — and I didn't notice how far I'd fallen until I could barely hear myself think.

The Hidden Decline No One Talks About

Here's the trap:

- You stop something you thought was holding you back.
- You feel clear for a while — powered by motivation, purpose, love.
- And then life piles on. Slowly. Quietly.
- The diet slips. The sleep breaks. The noise creeps in.
- You start caffeine. Add sugar. Chase dopamine.
- Then… meds. More pressure. Less support.
- And one day you wake up not okay — but you can't work out when it happened.

That's what happened to me.

And when everything collapsed — in mind, body, and spirit —

Cannabis was the first thing that came to mind.

Chapter 13 - Part 2

Back in Ibiza: The Moment of Clarity

I hadn't touched it in years.

But on that trip — raw, depleted, and stripped of who I was — I reached for something familiar. Something that used to soften the volume inside my head.

And I'm telling you now:

That moment didn't make me lazy.

It didn't make me "stoned."

It made me quiet.

It made me aware.

It made me, me — again.

Not permanently. Not magically. But... enough.

Enough to see that what I needed wasn't just rest — it was reset.

I had to come home to my mind — and I had to do it consciously.

Why It Helped Me — And Might Help Others Like Me

Let's be honest:

Cannabis isn't for everyone. It can make some people anxious, lazy, or numb.

But for me — a neurodivergent mind wired to overthink, hyperfocus, and burn out —

It created balance.

• It slowed the spin.
• Softened the pressure.
• Opened the window for reflection.
• Helped my sleep find rhythm again.
• And it made food choices clearer — because I could finally feel the difference.

I didn't realise until years later that I was likely self-medicating for ADHD and autistic traits without knowing it. It wasn't about "fun" — it was about function.

And that rebellious feeling?

That little dopamine boost from doing something "wrong"?

That probably helped too.

Because for people like us, rebellion sometimes feels like freedom.

Meds, Microdosing & Morning Flow

Today, I use both. Carefully.

- **A mild cannabis strain** — tiny amount, just in the morning, to soften the mental grip.
- **Lisdexamfetamine** — pulsed, not slammed. 20mg now. I used to be o n 70.
- **Natural movement, food, sunlight, rest.**

This combo works with my rhythm, not against it.

It doesn't silence me. It grounds me.

It doesn't blur the world. It sharpens it — in a way meds alone never could.

And more importantly, I listen now. To my body. My brain. My blood sugar. My emotions.

I track what shifts me up, down, or sideways.

And I use cannabis like a key — not a crutch.

Chapter 13 - Part 3

Let's Talk About Stigma, Science & Sanity

People will judge.

They'll assume you're lazy, addicted, and checked out.

But here's the truth:

- **Cannabis doesn't switch your life off — it can switch your perception back on.**
- **When used with intention, it can act as a mirror, a lens, or even a lifeline.**
- **Especially for neurodivergent people struggling to regulate overstimulation, insomnia, or executive function.**

We need better science.

Better understanding.

Better conversations.

Because when I finally saw what it was doing for me — not to me —

I realised it had been part of my toolkit all along.

Hidden behind shame.

Hidden behind society's rules.

But waiting patiently — like a soft light behind a curtain.

The Aha Moment: You Don't Know You're Lost Until You Stop Moving

I thought I was doing okay.

I was functioning. I was working. I was showing up.

But underneath it all, I was numb, dysregulated, and on autopilot.

It took cannabis to slow me down long enough to feel the mess I was in.

To grieve how far I'd slipped from clarity.

And to begin crawling back.

True recovery doesn't always look like strength.

Sometimes it looks like lying on a sofa, eyes closed, music on —

feeling your own breath for the first time in years.

And That's Why I Wrote This Book

Because if I can help one person pause before they spiral…

If I can help one parent or partner understand that cannabis isn't always a sign of giving up…

If I can help someone realise that clarity isn't just a goal — it's a feeling that can return…

Then every moment of this story was worth it.

You are not broken. You are not failing. You are not alone.

There is a version of you that's calm, clear, and awake.

And it's still in there. Waiting to be heard.

Let this be your moment —

To stop.
To breathe.
To reset.
To come home.

Key Takeaway:
Sometimes the path back to clarity isn't straight. And that's okay.

Beyond the Book – The Reset Program

The real magic happens when we connect.

That's why the Unboxed journey doesn't stop with a book. We're creating:

Local Reset Programs:

Courses led by real people who've walked the path — not influencers, not perfectionists.

But relatable humans. Trainers, chefs, ADHD mentors, breathwork teachers, and even massage therapists.

You pick your track. You build your version of clarity.

Outdoor Walks + Nature Time:

You don't heal in the place that made you sick.

So, we're bringing people outside again — to move, talk, and breathe.

Flexible Support:

Free for those in need. Funded through donations, grants, and our Give One model.

No guilt. No pressure. Just progress.

It's Not About Being Perfect. It's About Being Unboxed

I don't want you to become obsessed with food labels.

I don't want you to be afraid of every snack.

I just want you to see the system clearly enough to make real, conscious choices.

You can have clarity and chocolate.

You can be kind to your body without punishing yourself.

You can live a life with joy, not rules.

This isn't about turning your life upside down.

It's about finally flipping it right-side up.

Legacy Starts with You

If you've made it this far, then you've already started your legacy.

You're part of the movement now. Not a brand. Not a trend.

A clarity revolution.

And here's the best bit: You don't have to change the world alone.

You just have to light the next torch.

Let's do it together.

Let's get unboxed.

Key Takeaway:

Legacy isn't what you leave behind. It's what you pass forward.

From my family to your family. Thanks for picking this up.

Really. Whether you read one chapter or the whole lot — I appreciate you. This book came from a messy, painful place... but it gave me something back.

If it gave you something too — clarity, courage, curiosity — then it was worth every second.

Big thanks to the people who stood by me. To the health professionals who listened, explained, or even just showed interest. That mattered more than you know.

And if this sparked your journey...

Don't keep it to yourself. Let me know how it helped.

We're all still figuring this out. But we're doing it together.

Thanks,

Lee Jones

About the Author

Lee Jones is a business owner, father, and ADHD advocate from the Wirral. After years of struggling with brain fog, burnout, and feeling "different," he discovered how food additives and lifestyle choices were amplifying his symptoms.

Through his own journey of clarity, he founded the Unboxed movement — helping others escape the fog of processed living and return to their authentic selves.

When he's not writing or running his bespoke kitchen business, Kitch'en, Lee can be found building dens with his kids, planning his next business venture, or quietly advocating for a world where clarity isn't a luxury — it's a right.

This is his first book, but it may not be his last.

Resources & Next Steps

Want to continue your Unboxed journey?

- **Website:** [Coming Soon – www.unboxedtogrether.com]
- **App:** Unboxed additive tracker & wellness coach [In development]
- **Local Programs:** Reset courses in your area [Rolling out 2025]
- **Give One, Get One:** Help someone else start their journey
- **For Lee's kitchen business:** www.bespokekitch-en.co.uk

Remember: This book is based on personal experience and is not intended as medical advice. Please consult qualified professionals before making significant dietary or medical changes.

Quick additive guide

E102 – Tartrazine

Also known as: FD&C Yellow 5

Traffic Light Rating: Avoid 🔴

Side Effects:

· Hyperactivity (especially in children)

· Migraines and asthma in sensitive individuals

Interaction Warning:

· May worsen symptoms when combined with sodium benzoate (E211)

E110 – Sunset Yellow FCF

Also known as: FD&C Yellow 6

Traffic Light Rating: Avoid 🔴

Side Effects:

· Linked to skin rashes, abdominal pain, hyperactivity

Interaction Warning:

· Effects may intensify alongside other azo dyes (e.g. E104, E122)

E120 – Cochineal

Also known as: Carminic acid, Carmines

Traffic Light Rating: Caution 🟡

Side Effects:

· Allergic reactions (especially in asthmatics)

· Rare anaphylaxis cases

Interaction Warning:

· Can compound allergy risk with other natural dyes (e.g. E160b)

E211 – Sodium Benzoate

Also known as: Benzoate of soda

Traffic Light Rating: Avoid 🔴

Side Effects:

· Linked to hyperactivity, cell damage

· Potential formation of benzene (a carcinogen)

Interaction Warning:

· Forms benzene when combined with ascorbic acid (E300)

E220 – Sulphur Dioxide

Also known as: Sulfurous acid anhydride

Traffic Light Rating: Avoid 🔴

Side Effects:

· Asthma attacks, hives, nausea

Interaction Warning:

· High-risk when paired with other sulphites (E221–E228)

E250 – Sodium Nitrite

Also known as: —

Traffic Light Rating: Avoid 🔴

Side Effects:

· Linked to bowel cancer

· Headaches, low blood pressure

Interaction Warning:

· Forms carcinogenic nitrosamines when heated with proteins

E951 – Aspartame

Also known as: NutraSweet, Equal

Traffic Light Rating: Avoid 🔴

Side Effects:

· Headaches, anxiety, seizures in sensitive individuals

· Dangerous for people with PKU

Interaction Warning:

· May amplify side effects when combined with MSG (E621)

E104 – Quinoline Yellow

Also known as: CI 47005

Traffic Light Rating: Avoid 🔴

Side Effects:

· Linked to hyperactivity and behaviour issues

· May cause skin rashes or digestive upset

Interaction Warning:

· Can intensify effects when combined with other azo dyes (E102, E110)

E122 – Azorubine

Also known as: Carmoisine

Traffic Light Rating: Avoid 🔴

Side Effects:

· May cause hyperactivity, asthma, and allergic skin reactions

Interaction Warning:

· Effects compounded with other red azo dyes (e.g. E124, E129)

E124 – Ponceau 4R

Also known as: Cochineal Red A

Traffic Light Rating: Avoid 🔴

Side Effects:

· Associated with cancer in animal studies

· Triggers allergic reactions and asthma

Interaction Warning:

· Often found with sodium benzoate (E211), which increases risk

E129 – Allura Red AC

Also known as: FD&C Red 40

Traffic Light Rating: Avoid 🔴

Side Effects:

· May trigger ADHD symptoms

· Linked to allergic reactions, especially in aspirin-sensitive people

Interaction Warning:

· May interact with E211 and E102 to intensify behaviour effects

E133 – Brilliant Blue FCF

Also known as: FD&C Blue 1

Traffic Light Rating: Caution 🟡

Side Effects:

· May cause allergic skin or respiratory reactions

Interaction Warning:

· Caution when used with other synthetic dyes

E150c – Ammonia Caramel

Also known as: Caramel Colour III

Traffic Light Rating: Caution 🟡

Side Effects:

· May increase cancer risk in high doses

· Some studies suggest effects on immune health

Interaction Warning:

· Heat processing can generate 4-MEI, a possible carcinogen

E160b – Annatto

Also known as: Bixin, Norbixin

Traffic Light Rating: Caution 🟡

Side Effects:

· Can cause hives and swelling

· Rare cases of irritable bowel reactions

Interaction Warning:

· May heighten allergic response if combined with E120 (Cochineal)

E200 – Sorbic Acid

Also known as: —

Traffic Light Rating: Caution 🟡

Side Effects:

· Skin and eye irritation

· May worsen asthma in sensitive individuals

Interaction Warning:

· Can interact with sulphites (E220–E228) to increase
  respiratory symptoms

E202 – Potassium Sorbate

Also known as: —

Traffic Light Rating: Caution 🟡

Side Effects:

· May cause migraines and allergic reactions

· Linked to skin irritation when used in cosmetics

Interaction Warning:

· Potential synergy with benzoates or sulphites in triggering allergies

E210 – Benzoic Acid

Also known as: —

Traffic Light Rating: Avoid 🔴

Side Effects:

· Can irritate skin, eyes, and lungs

· May worsen behavioural symptoms in children

Interaction Warning:

· Forms carcinogenic benzene when mixed with vitamin C (E300)

E221 – Sodium Sulphite

Also known as: —

Traffic Light Rating: Avoid 🔴

Side Effects:

· Triggers asthma, wheezing, and nausea

· May cause skin hives in sulphite-sensitive individuals

Interaction Warning:

· Enhanced respiratory effects when combined with E220 or E228

E250 – Sodium Nitrite

Also known as: —

Traffic Light Rating: Avoid 🔴

Side Effects:

· Strongly linked to bowel cancer

· Can cause headaches, dizziness, and blood pressure drops

Interaction Warning:

· Forms nitrosamines (a known carcinogen) when cooked
  with proteins

E251 – Sodium Nitrate

Also known as: —

Traffic Light Rating: Avoid 🔴

Side Effects:

· Risk of blue baby syndrome in infants

· Associated with gastric and colon cancers

Interaction Warning:

· Converts to nitrite in the body, triggering same risks as E250

E260 – Acetic Acid

Also known as: Vinegar acid

Traffic Light Rating: Safe 🟢

Side Effects:

· May irritate throat or stomach in high doses

Interaction Warning:

· Generally safe, but may increase acidity effects with other
  acidic additives

E300 – Ascorbic Acid

Also known as: Vitamin C

Traffic Light Rating: Safe 🟢

Side Effects:

· Generally safe, though large doses may cause mild stomach upset

Interaction Warning:

· Can react with benzoates (e.g. E211) to form benzene — a
  known carcinogen

E322 – Lecithins

Also known as: —

Traffic Light Rating: Safe 🟢

Side Effects:

· May trigger soy allergy in sensitive individuals

Interaction Warning:

· Watch for allergens when derived from GMO soy or egg sources

E330 – Citric Acid

Also known as: —

Traffic Light Rating: Safe 🟢

Side Effects:

· Mouth and stomach irritation in large quantities

Interaction Warning:

· Can contribute to benzene formation if paired with E211
  (Sodium Benzoate)

E338 – Phosphoric Acid

Also known as: —

Traffic Light Rating: Caution 🟡

Side Effects:

· May reduce bone mineral density with high intake

Interaction Warning:

· Can worsen calcium/magnesium depletion if overused with acidic preservatives

E400 – Alginic Acid

Also known as: —

Traffic Light Rating: Safe 🟢

Side Effects:

· Rare digestive upset in high doses

Interaction Warning:

· Safe, minimal interaction risk

E412 – Guar Gum

Also known as: —

Traffic Light Rating: Caution 🟡

Side Effects:

· Bloating, gas, or loose stools in some individuals

Interaction Warning:

· May affect medication absorption in sensitive people when taken in large amounts

E415 – Xanthan Gum

Also known as: —

Traffic Light Rating Caution 🟡

Side Effects:

· Bloating, diarrhoea, or gas

· May cause issues for those with corn allergies

Interaction Warning:

· Can interact with other thickening agents to increase gut irritation

E471 – Mono- and Diglycerides of Fatty Acids

Also known as: —

Traffic Light Rating: Caution 🟡

Side Effects:

· May be derived from animal or GMO soy sources

· Possible trans fats if highly processed

Interaction Warning:

· Unclear origin can complicate allergen tracking (soy, dairy, etc.)

E466 – Carboxymethylcellulose

Also known as: CMC

Traffic Light Rating: Caution 🟡

Side Effects:

· Can disrupt gut lining and microbiota balance

Interaction Warning:

· Gut irritation may be worsened when combined with emulsifiers like E471

E950 – Acesulfame K

Also known as: Acesulfame Potassium

Traffic Light Rating: Avoid 🔴

Side Effects:

· Linked to thyroid disruption in animal studies

· May have bitter aftertaste and affect appetite hormones

Interaction Warning:

· Often used with other sweeteners (E951, E955), compounding risk

E951 – Aspartame

Also known as: NutraSweet, Equal

Traffic Light Rating: Avoid 🔴

Side Effects:

· Headaches, mood swings, anxiety

· Unsafe for people with PKU (phenylketonuria)

Interaction Warning:

· May amplify neurological effects when combined with caffeine or
  MSG (E621)

E952 – Cyclamic Acid and Its Salts

Also known as: Cyclamates

Traffic Light Rating: Avoid 🔴

Side Effects:

· Banned in US over cancer concerns

· May cause bladder damage in long-term animal studies

Interaction Warning:

· Often blended with other synthetic sweeteners — cumulative
  effect unclear

E954 – Saccharin

Also known as: Sweet'N Low

Traffic Light Rating: Avoid 🔴

Side Effects:

· Linked to cancer in rats (controversial in humans)

· Can alter gut microbiome

Interaction Warning:

· Avoid stacking with other sweeteners due to unclear combined risk

E955 – Sucralose

Also known as: Splenda

Traffic Light Rating: Caution 🟡

Side Effects:

· May harm beneficial gut bacteria

· Can form harmful compounds when heated

Interaction Warning:

· Avoid baking or combining with high heat — toxic byproducts
  may form

E999 – Quillaia Extract

Also known as: Quillaja saponaria extract

Traffic Light Rating: Caution 🟡

Side Effects:

· May cause nausea, digestive discomfort

· Possible interaction with heart medications

Interaction Warning:

· Contains natural saponins; can interact with other
  active compounds

E320 – Butylated Hydroxyanisole (BHA)

Also known as: —

Traffic Light Rating: Avoid 🔴

Side Effects:

· Suspected human carcinogen

· Can disrupt hormone function

Interaction Warning:

· Often paired with BHT (E321), compounding long-term toxicity

E321 – Butylated Hydroxytoluene (BHT)

Also known as: —

Traffic Light Rating: Avoid 🔴

Side Effects:

· Linked to liver and kidney stress in animals

· May impair immune response

Interaction Warning:

· Long-term use alongside E320 (BHA) may increase cumulative risk

E385 – Calcium Disodium EDTA

Also known as: EDTA

Traffic Light Rating: Caution 🟡

Side Effects:

· Can cause digestive issues

· Binds minerals and may affect nutrient absorption

Interaction Warning:

· Avoid excess intake with mineral supplements —
  interference possible

E153 – Vegetable Carbon

Also known as: Activated charcoal

Traffic Light Rating: Safe 🟢

Side Effects:

· Minimal, but may cause black stool or mild GI upset

Interaction Warning:

· Can reduce absorption of medication when consumed together

E524 – Sodium Hydroxide

Also known as: Caustic soda

Traffic Light Rating: Caution 🟡

Side Effects:

· Corrosive in raw form, but safe in trace food processing

Interaction Warning:

· Residuals unlikely but should not be consumed in pure form

E535 – Sodium Ferrocyanide

Also known as: —

Traffic Light Rating: Caution 🟡

Side Effects:

· Considered safe at low levels

· High doses could release cyanide in acidic conditions (rare)

Interaction Warning:

· Avoid concentrated exposure with acidic preservatives

E586 – 4-Hexylresorcinol

Also known as: —

Traffic Light Rating: Avoid 🔴

Side Effects:

· Potential endocrine disruptor

· Data limited but early concern exists

Interaction Warning:

· Best avoided alongside other hormone-disrupting additives

E620 – Glutamic Acid

Also known as: —

Traffic Light Rating: Caution 🟡

Side Effects:

· Can trigger MSG-like symptoms (headaches, flushing) in sensitive people

· May cause excitability or gut discomfort

Interaction Warning:

· Effects heightened when paired with E621 (MSG), E627, or E631

E621 – Monosodium Glutamate (MSG)

Also known as: Flavour enhancer 621

Traffic Light Rating: Caution 🟡

Side Effects:

· Headaches, sweating, chest tightness in some individuals ("Chinese restaurant syndrome")

Interaction Warning:

· Often combined with E627 and E631, which can intensify effects

E627 – Disodium Guanylate

Also known as: —

Traffic Light Rating: Caution 🟡

Side Effects:

· Not recommended for young children or asthmatics

· May cause flushing or itching

Interaction Warning:

· Enhances effects of E621 (MSG) and should not be used alone

E631 – Disodium Inosinate

Also known as: —

Traffic Light Rating: Caution 🟡

Side Effects:

· May trigger purine reactions (avoid in gout)

· Can cause nausea or dizziness

Interaction Warning:

· Works synergistically with MSG (E621) and E627

E635 – Disodium 5'-ribonucleotides

Also known as: Mix of E627 + E631

Traffic Light Rating: Caution 🟡

Side Effects:

· Can cause rashes and headaches

· Unsuitable for infants or those with asthma

Interaction Warning:

· Strong flavour enhancer combo — effects compounded with MSG (E621)

E928 – Benzoyl Peroxide

Also known as: —

Traffic Light Rating: Avoid 🔴

Side Effects:

· Possible allergen; used to bleach flour

· Can irritate skin and mucous membranes

Interaction Warning:

· Oxidising agent — avoid combining with reducing or acidic additives

E507 – Hydrochloric Acid

Also known as: —

Traffic Light Rating: Caution 🟡

Side Effects:

· Corrosive in pure form; safe in trace food processing

Interaction Warning:

· Incompatible with alkaline preservatives or metal compounds

E510 – Ammonium Chloride

Also known as: Salmiak

Traffic Light Rating: Caution 🟡

Side Effects:

· Can cause nausea and muscle weakness in excess

· High doses may disrupt electrolyte balance

Interaction Warning:

· Avoid combining with sodium-rich preservatives or diuretics

E1422 – Acetylated Distarch Adipate

Also known as: Modified starch

Traffic Light Rating: Caution 🟡

Side Effects:

· Limited human data; may cause digestive upset

· Often GMO-derived

Interaction Warning:

· May slow medication absorption if consumed in large quantities

E1442 – Hydroxypropyl Distarch Phosphate

Also known as: Modified starch

Traffic Light Rating: Caution 🟡

Side Effects:

· Can cause bloating or gas

· Limited long-term safety data

Interaction Warning:

· Potential cumulative effect when used with other starch
  modifiers (E1450)

E1450 – Starch Sodium Octenyl Succinate

Also known as: Modified starch

Traffic Light Rating: Caution 🟡

Side Effects:

· May affect gut health in some people

· Often used in infant formula — controversial

Interaction Warning:

· Not suitable for babies under 12 weeks due to digestion impact

E551 – Silicon Dioxide

Also known as: Silica

Traffic Light Rating: Safe 🟢

Side Effects:

· Minimal — may cause gut irritation in ultra-processed forms

Interaction Warning:

· Safe alone, but watch for nanoparticle versions in supplements

E150d – Sulphite Ammonia Caramel

Also known as: Caramel Colour IV

Traffic Light Rating: Caution 🟡

Side Effects:

· May contain 4-MEI, a suspected carcinogen

· Can trigger asthma in sensitive individuals

Interaction Warning:

· Combined with caffeine (in colas) may stress the liver

E160a – Beta-Carotene

Also known as: Provitamin A

Traffic Light Rating: Safe 🟢

Side Effects:

· Generally safe; very high doses may colour skin orange

Interaction Warning:

· Antioxidant effects may diminish when paired with
  heavy preservatives

E161g – Canthaxanthin

Also known as: —

Traffic Light Rating: Avoid 🔴

Side Effects:

· Linked to eye and liver damage at high doses

Interaction Warning:

· May increase oxidative stress when used with other
  artificial colourants

E200–E203 – Sorbates Group (Summary)

Includes: E200 Sorbic Acid, E202 Potassium Sorbate,
E203 Calcium Sorbate

Traffic Light Rating: Caution 🟡

Side Effects:

· May cause skin irritation, asthma, or migraines

Interaction Warning:

· Enhanced effects when combined with benzoates or sulphites

E300–E304 – Ascorbates Group (Summary)

Includes: E300 Ascorbic Acid, E301 Sodium Ascorbate, E302 Calcium
Ascorbate, E304 Fatty Acid Esters

Traffic Light Rating: Safe 🟢

Side Effects:

· Generally beneficial (vitamin C forms)

· May cause minor GI issues in high doses

Interaction Warning:

· When mixed with benzoates (e.g. E211), can form benzene —
  a carcinogen

E407 – Carrageenan

Also known as: Irish Moss Extract

Traffic Light Rating: Avoid 🔴

Side Effects:

· Linked to gut inflammation and ulcers in some studies

· Can cause bloating or IBS-like symptoms

Interaction Warning:

· May worsen gut barrier issues when combined with emulsifiers
  (E466, E471)

E414 – Acacia Gum

Also known as: Gum Arabic

Traffic Light Rating: Safe 🟢

Side Effects:

· Mild gas or bloating in sensitive individuals

Interaction Warning:

· Generally safe unless used with other fermentable fibres (FODMAPs)

E432 – Polysorbate 20

Also known as: —

Traffic Light Rating: Avoid 🔴

Side Effects:

· Can weaken gut barrier and alter microbiota

· May trigger skin or eye irritation

Interaction Warning:

· Avoid combining with E433, E435, or other polysorbates —
  cumulative gut effects

E433 – Polysorbate 80

Also known as: Tween 80

Traffic Light Rating: Avoid 🔴

Side Effects:

· Linked to fertility disruption and gut inflammation in mice

· May affect immune response

Interaction Warning:

· May increase uptake of other harmful substances across the gut wall

E450 – Diphosphates

Also known as: Disodium diphosphate, tetrasodium diphosphate

Traffic Light Rating: Caution 🟡

Side Effects:

· May disturb calcium absorption and kidney health

Interaction Warning:

· Not recommended for people with kidney disease or children
  in excess

E471 – Mono-and Diglycerides of Fatty Acids

Also known as: —

Traffic Light Rating: Caution 🟡

Side Effects:

· May contain hidden trans fats

· Can be derived from animal or GMO soy sources

Interaction Warning:

· Gut interaction risk when combined with emulsifiers like E472

E472 – Acetic/Lactic/Citric Esters of Mono- and Diglycerides

Also known as: —

Traffic Light Rating: Caution 🟡

Side Effects:

· Possible allergen trace residues from manufacturing

· Poorly tolerated in some with IBS

Interaction Warning:

· May increase food chemical sensitivity when combined with other emulsifiers

E473 – Sucrose Esters of Fatty Acids

Also known as: Sugar esters

Traffic Light Rating: Caution 🟡

Side Effects:

· Generally low risk, but may cause loose stools in high doses

Interaction Warning:

· Watch for gut irritation when combined with other emulsifiers like E471 or E472

E481 – Sodium Stearoyl Lactylate

Also known as: SSL

Traffic Light Rating: Caution 🟡

Side Effects:

· May cause nausea or diarrhoea in sensitive individuals

Interaction Warning:

· Can exacerbate gut sensitivity when paired with synthetic dough conditioners

E482 – Calcium Stearoyl Lactylate

Also known as: CSL

Traffic Light Rating: Caution 🟡

Side Effects:

· Similar to E481; may alter gut flora

Interaction Warning:

· Often used with emulsifiers and whiteners — can increase gut strain

E491 – Sorbitan Monostearate

Also known as: —

Traffic Light Rating: Caution 🟡

Side Effects:

· May cause mild laxative effect

Interaction Warning:

· Effects may intensify with other sorbitan or polysorbate compounds

E492 – Sorbitan Tristearate

Also known as: —

Traffic Light Rating: Caution 🟡

Side Effects:

· Generally tolerated, though may cause digestive discomfort

Interaction Warning:

· Works similarly to E491 — increased effect if combined

E500 – Sodium Carbonates

Also known as: Baking soda, washing soda

Traffic Light Rating: Safe 🟢

Side Effects:

· In high amounts, may cause alkalinity-related issues

Interaction Warning:

· Safe when used properly; avoid mixing with strong acids outside food

E508 – Potassium Chloride

Also known as: Salt substitute

Traffic Light Rating: Caution 🟡

Side Effects:

· May affect heart rhythm in high doses

· Can taste metallic

Interaction Warning:

· Avoid high doses with potassium-sparing medications or kidney issues

E620–E635 – Flavour Enhancer Group (Summary)

Includes: MSG, Disodium Inosinate, Guanylate, 5'-ribonucleotides

Traffic Light Rating: Caution 🟡

Side Effects:

· Headaches, flushing, gut sensitivity

Interaction Warning:

· Stronger when combined — often found in savoury snacks and instant noodles

E951 – Aspartame

Also known as: NutraSweet, Equal

Traffic Light Rating: Avoid 🔴

Side Effects:

· Headaches, mood swings, dizziness

· Unsafe for people with PKU

Interaction Warning:

· Effects amplified when used with caffeine or MSG (E621)

E955 – Sucralose

Also known as: Splenda

Traffic Light Rating: Caution 🟡

Side Effects:

· May disrupt gut microbiota

· Toxic when heated (forms chloropropanols)

Interaction Warning:

· Avoid baking with it or mixing with acidic preservatives

E965 – Maltitol

Also known as: —

Traffic Light Rating: Caution 🟡

Side Effects:

· Bloating, gas, diarrhoea in high amounts

Interaction Warning:

· Effect intensified when combined with other polyols (
  e.g. E420, E968)

E966 – Lactitol
Also known as: —
Traffic Light Rating: Caution 🟡
Side Effects:
· Can cause bloating, cramps, and flatulence
Interaction Warning:
· Similar to E965 — cumulative laxative effect

E967 – Xylitol
Also known as: —
Traffic Light Rating: Caution 🟡
Side Effects:
· Mild laxative effect at high doses
Interaction Warning:
· Dangerous to dogs — caution with children handling products
  around pets

E968 – Erythritol
Also known as: —
Traffic Light Rating: Caution 🟡
Side Effects:
· Generally well tolerated; may cause mild digestive upset
Interaction Warning:
· May combine with other polyols to increase effect

E999 – Quillaia Extract

Also known as: Soapbark extract

Traffic Light Rating: Caution 🟡

Side Effects:

· Nausea, GI irritation in high doses

Interaction Warning:

· Avoid combining with immune-sensitising compounds

E1200 – Polydextrose

Also known as: —

Traffic Light Rating: Caution 🟡

Side Effects:

· Gas, bloating, and loose stools

Interaction Warning:

· Often combined with artificial sweeteners — may intensify
  side effects

E1400–1450 – Modified Starches (Summary)

Includes: E1400–E1450 group

Traffic Light Rating: Caution 🟡

Side Effects:

· Possible allergen traces

· May affect digestion if overused

Interaction Warning:

· Often found with thickeners and emulsifiers — may slow
  nutrient absorption

E1520 – Propylene Glycol

Also known as: —

Traffic Light Rating: Avoid 🔴

Side Effects:

· Can cause kidney or liver issues in high doses

· Known irritant in cosmetics

Interaction Warning:

· Often found in vape liquids, food flavourings — toxic if combined
with alcohol

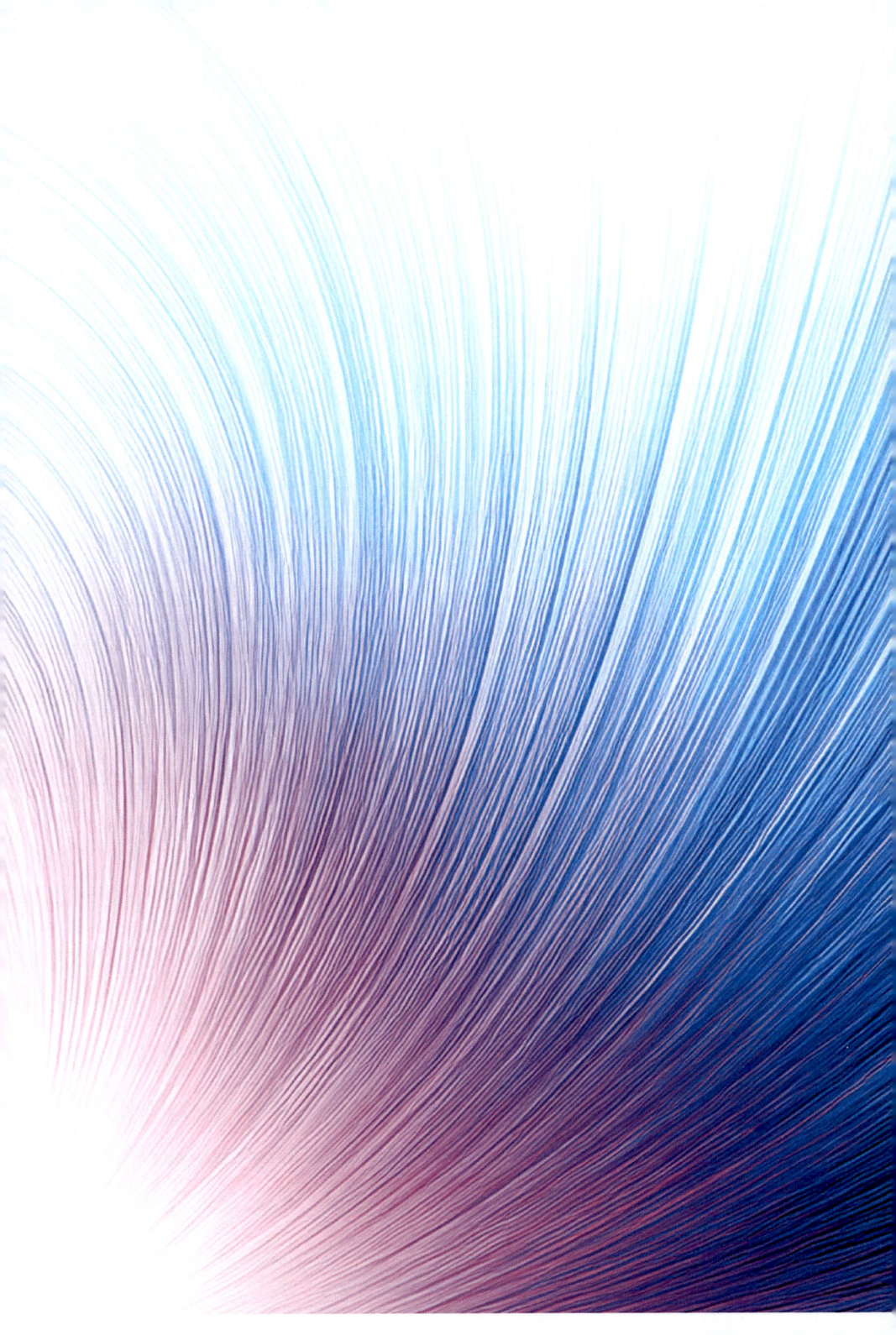

www.ingramcontent.com/pod-product-compliance
Lightning Source LLC
Chambersburg PA
CBRC091536260326
41914CB00020B/1634